The Right Ventricle in Adults with Tetralogy of Fallot

Massimo Chessa • Alessandro Giamberti
Editors

The Right Ventricle in Adults with Tetralogy of Fallot

Foreword by Gary D. Webb

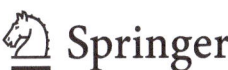 Springer

Massimo Chessa
IRCCS Policlinico San Donato
Pediatric and Adult
Congenital Heart Center
San Donato Milanese (Mi)
Italy

Alessandro Giamberti
IRCCS Policlinico San Donato
Cardio-Thoracic Surgery
San Donato Milanese (Mi)
Italy

ISBN 978-88-470-2357-4

ISBN 978-88-470-2358-1 (eBook)

DOI 10.1007/978-88-470-2358-1

Springer Milan Dordrecht Heidelberg London New York

Library of Congress Control Number: 2012930654

5 4 3 2 1

2012   2013   2014

Cover design: eStudio Calamar S.L.
Typesetting: Graphostudio, Milan, Italy

Springer-Verlag Italia S.r.l. – Via Decembrio 28 – I-20137 Milan
Springer is a part of Springer Science+Business Media (www.springer.com)

Foreword

Do we need a textbook on the right ventricle in adults with tetralogy of Fallot? Surely those of us who look after these patients are well-informed about all the issues in their assessment and care! Yet, as it turns out, not to the extent we imagined. In this volume Massimo Chessa and Alessandro Giamberti concisely and effectively encourage us to think more deeply about these patients and how we might best understand their problems such that we are able to offer them the best possible chance of long-term good health.

In an excellent chapter on the anatomy of tetralogy of Fallot, the authors describe the unique anatomical relationships, as inferred from cardiac specimens at the University of Padua. This is most instructive and so are the sizable number of excellent photographs used to support the text.

In a stimulating chapter on the genetics of tetralogy of Fallot, the authors focus in on 22Q11 deletion syndrome. While noting that it is diagnosed in about 10% of such patients, they point out that with the new molecular technique of comparative genomic hybridization microchromosomal anomalies have been identified in 21% of tetralogy of Fallot patients: NKX 2.5 mutations in up to 4% of nonsyndromic tetralogy patients, CITED2 mutations in 6% of tetralogy patients, and JAG1 in about 3%. They also note that tetralogy, when associated with trisomy 21, is characterized by a large ventricular septal defect (VSD) and adequately sized pulmonary arteries (PAs). By contrast, in patients with tetralogy and 22Q11 deletion syndrome, the phenotype includes anomalies of the aortic arch, PAs, infundibular septum, and pulmonary valve.

The next chapter is a fascinating one, focusing on stem cells and the right ventricle. In their fascinating state-of-the-art review of this topic, the authors make the case that both tetralogy and arrhythmogenic right ventricular cardiomyopathy can be seen as diseases of stem cells.

In the chapter on the pathophysiology of tetralogy, the authors begin with a stimulating review of the embryology of the right ventricle, highlighting the importance of the secondary heart field in this respect and in the normal embryogenesis of the cardiac outflow tract. They also consider the differences in the timing of left and right ventricular myocardium development, thus offering a basis for the differential expression of developmental abnormalities. According to evidence reviewed by the authors, the ability of the right ventricular myocardium to adapt to chronic hypoxia is impaired in patients with tetralogy of Fallot. By contrast, the left ventricle, through the hypoxia-induced-factor (HIF-1) pathway, has several mechanisms to accommodate severe hypoxia. These principles provide a means of better understanding long-term right ventricular myocardial failure in patients with cyanotic congenital heart disease.

In a very comprehensive chapter on the use of echocardiography in patients with tetralogy, the results of 3-D echocardiography and cardiac magnetic resonance are compared. While 3-D echo allows a better assessment of pulmonary valve morphology, it underestimates right ventricular volumes and ejection fractions, especially with larger volumes.

There is a separate chapter on the timing of right ventricular outflow tract management in tetralogy patients with pulmonary regurgitation. The authors comment on the absence of reliable studies to help clinicians determine when intervention for significant pulmonary regurgitation will be most effective. They correctly observe that it is not yet clear whether a full normalization of right ventricular volumes is required to improve the long-term outcomes of these patients. Their comparison of the American, Canadian, and European guidelines on this topic are accompanied by the inclusion criteria for pulmonary valve replacement used at the German Heart Center in Munich.

Not surprisingly, there is a chapter on the percutaneous pulmonary valve. The authors point out that failing conduits are rarely circular and have complex shapes and stenoses. Given these challenges, the Melody valve remains competent in different sizes and geometries. Its size limitation (22 mm) is overcome by the Edwards Sapien valve, the major indication of which is the treatment of larger conduits (up to 25 mm). According to the authors, the stent fracture rate can be substantially reduced by implanting one or more stents within the conduit until it is "prepared" for placement of the Melody valve.

A separate chapter focuses on the management of residual VSDs and branch pulmonary artery stenosis in the catheterization laboratory. The latter condition has been reported in as many as 17% of patients with tetralogy, especially involving the left PA. Indications for intervention are thoughtfully presented. The authors indicate a preference for stenting branch PA stenoses in adult patients, commenting that they do not use self-expanding stents because of the inability to redilate them. While making a good case for interventional catheter closure of residual VSDs, the authors also acknowledge the potential value of a hybrid approach in which the VSD is closed through a midline sternotomy, avoiding cardiopulmonary bypass by introducing a device through the right ventricle.

In their chapter on surgical pulmonary valve implantation, the authors review the various types of valves that can be used for this purpose. After an extensive survey of the literature, they provide a variety of reasons for their preferred approach to pulmonary valve replacement, using stented bioprosthetic valves. The references provided in relation to this discussion are well worth exploring.

Surgical procedures performed in the course of redo procedures on tetralogy patients are discussed in another chapter. In a series from Milan, 80% of patients who underwent pulmonary valve replacement had additional procedures, the most frequent of which were right ventricular remodeling, tricuspid valve repair, and arrhythmia surgery. In the authors' opinion, this experience supports the contention that surgery on these patients had probably been left until too late. While ascending aortic dilation is common in tetralogy patients, the risk of aortic dissection or even progressive dilation is low.

The book concludes with chapters on late arrhythmias and on the perioperative management of the right ventricle.

Overall, this excellent source of information and discussion will stimulate cardiologists and surgeons interested in the adult tetralogy patient to think beyond the frequently narrow limits of our assumptions and to begin to appreciate in a more complex and scientific manner the challenges these patients present.

It is my pleasure and privilege to warmly recommend this text to you, my colleagues.

March 2012   Gary D. Webb, M.D.
                                              Cincinnati Children's Hospital Heart Institute

Contents

1   **Introduction** 1
Massimo Chessa and Alessandro Giamberti

2   **Anatomy of Tetralogy of Fallot** 3
Carla Frescura and Gaetano Thiene

3   **Genetics** 27
M. Cristina Digilio, Bruno Dallapiccola and Bruno Marino

4   **Stem Cells and the Right Ventricle** 39
Luigi Anastasia and Marco Piccoli

5   **Pathophysiology in Tetralogy of Fallot** 47
Gabriele Egidy Assenza and Michael J. Landzberg

6   **Tetralogy of Fallot: Late Outcome** 61
Jochen Weil

7   **Tetralogy of Fallot: The Failing Right Ventricle** 75
Folkert J. Meijboom and Barbara Mulder

8   **Imaging Evaluation** 91
Claudio Bussadori

9   **Timing for RVOT Management** 113
Harald Kaemmerer, Andreas Eicken and John Hess

10 **Percutaneous Pulmonary Valve** 125
Mark S. Turner, Mario Carminati and Philipp Bonhoeffer

11   **Other Transcatheter Procedures** 133
     Massimo Chessa and Gianfranco Butera

12   **Surgical Pulmonary Valve Implantation** 145
     Alessandro Giamberti, Giuseppe Pomè and Alessandro Frigiola

13   **Other Surgical Procedures** 155
     Alessandro Giamberti

14   **Late Arrhythmias: Current Approaches** 167
     Sara Foresti, Maria Cristina Tavera, Pierpaolo Lupo
     and Riccardo Cappato

15   **Perioperative Right Ventricular Management** 179
     Marco Ranucci

Contributors

Luigi Anastasia Department of Medical Chemistry, Biochemistry and Biotechnology, University of Milan, Italy; IRCCS Policlinico San Donato, San Donato Milanese (Mi), Italy

Philipp Bonhoeffer Fondazione Toscana Gabriele Monasterio, CNR, Pisa, Italy

Claudio Bussadori IRCCS Policlinico San Donato, Pediatric and Adult Congenital Heart Center, San Donato Milanese (Mi), Italy

Gianfranco Butera IRCCS Policlinico San Donato, Pediatric and Adult Congenital Heart Center, San Donato Milanese (Mi), Italy

Riccardo Cappato IRCCS Policlinico San Donato, Arrhythmia and Electrophysiology Center, San Donato Milanese (Mi), Italy

Mario Carminati IRCCS Policlinico San Donato, Pediatric and Adult Congenital Heart Center, San Donato Milanese (Mi), Italy

Massimo Chessa IRCCS Policlinico San Donato, Pediatric and Adult Congenital Heart Center, San Donato Milanese (Mi), Italy

Bruno Dallapiccola Medical Genetics, Bambino Gesù Pediatric Hospital, IRCCS, Rome, Italy

M. Cristina Digilio Medical Genetics, Bambino Gesù Pediatric Hospital, IRCCS, Rome, Italy

Gabriele Egidy Assenza Boston Adult Congenital Heart and Pulmonary Hypertension Program, Children's Hospital Boston, Brigham and Women's Hospital, Harvard Medical School, Boston, MA, USA; Department of Clinical and Molecular Medicine, Sant'Andrea Hospital, Sapienza University, Rome, Italy

Andreas Eicken Department of Pediatric Cardiology and Congenital Heart Disease, German Heart Center, Technical University of Munich, Munich, Germany

Sara Foresti IRCCS Policlinico San Donato, Arrhythmia and Electrophysiology Center, San Donato Milanese (Mi), Italy

Carla Frescura Department of Cardiological, Thoracic and Vascular Sciences, University of Padua, Padua, Italy

Alessandro Frigiola IRCCS Policlinico San Donato, Cardio-Thoracic Surgery, San Donato Milanese (Mi), Italy

Alessandro Giamberti IRCCS Policlinico San Donato, Cardio-Thoracic Surgery, San Donato Milanese (Mi), Italy

John Hess Department of Pediatric Cardiology and Congenital Heart Disease, German Heart Center, Technical University of Munich, Munich, Germany

Harald Kaemmerer Department of Pediatric Cardiology and Congenital Heart Disease, German Heart Center, Technical University of Munich, Munich, Germany

Michael J. Landzberg Boston Adult Congenital Heart and Pulmonary Hypertension Program, Children's Hospital Boston, Brigham and Women's Hospital, Harvard Medical School, Boston, MA, USA

Pierpaolo Lupo IRCCS Policlinico San Donato, Arrhythmia and Electrophysiology Center, San Donato Milanese (Mi), Italy

Bruno Marino Pediatric Cardiology, Department of Pediatrics, Sapienza University, Rome, Italy

Folkert J. Meijboom Departments of Cardiology and Pediatric Cardiology, University Medical Center Utrecht, Utrecht, The Netherlands

Barbara Mulder Department of Cardiology, Amsterdam Medical Center University of Amsterdam, Amsterdam, The Netherlands

Marco Piccoli IRCCS Policlinico San Donato, San Donato Milanese (MI), Italy

Giuseppe Pomè IRCCS Policlinico San Donato, Cardio-Thoracic Surgery, San Donato Milanese (Mi), Italy

Marco Ranucci IRCCS Policlinico San Donato, Cardio-Thoracic Anesthesia and ICU, San Donato Milanese (Mi), Italy

Maria Cristina Tavera IRCCS Policlinico San Donato, Arrhythmia and Electrophysiology Center, San Donato Milanese (Mi), Italy

Gaetano Thiene Department of Cardiological, Thoracic and Vascular Sciences, University of Padua, Padua, Italy

Mark S. Turner Department of Cardiology, Bristol Heart Institute, Bristol, UK

Jochen Weil Department of Pediatric Cardiology, University Heart Center Hamburg, Hamburg, Germany

Abbreviations

ACE	angiotensin-converting enzyme
AP	angina pectoris
APC	atriopulmonary connection
AR	aortic regurgitation
AS	aortic stenosis
ASD	atrial septal defect
AV	atrioventricular
AVA	aortic valve area
AVSD	atrioventricular septal defect
BAV	bicuspid aortic valve
BNP	B-type natriuretic peptide
BSA	body surface area
CAD	coronary artery disease
ccTGA	congenitally corrected transposition of the great arteries
CHD	congenital heart disease
CMR	cardiac magnetic resonance
CoA	coarctation of the aorta
CPET	cardiopulmonary exercise testing
CRT	cardiac resynchronization therapy
CT	computed tomography
DCRV	double-chambered right ventricle
ECG	electrocardiogram
EF	ejection fraction
EP	electrophysiology
ERA	endothelin receptor antagonist
FISH	fluorescent *in situ* hybridization
GUCH	grown-up congenital heart disease
ICD	implantable cardioverter defibrillator
IE	infective endocarditis
INR	international normalized ratio
IVC	inferior vena cava

LA	left atrium
LPA	left pulmonary artery
L-R shunt	left-to-right shunt
LV	left ventricle
LVEF	left ventricular ejection fraction
LVESD	left ventricular end-systolic diameter
LVH	left ventricular hypertrophy
LVOT	left ventricular outflow tract
LVOTO	left ventricular outflow tract obstruction
MAPCAs	major aortic pulmonary collaterals
MCV	mean corpuscular volume
NYHA	New York Heart Association
PA	pulmonary artery
PA + VSD	pulmonary atresia with ventricular septal defect
PAH	pulmonary arterial hypertension
PAP	pulmonary artery pressure
PDA	patent ductus arteriosus
PFO	patent foramen ovale
PLE	protein-losing enteropathy
PM	pacemaker
PPVI	percutaneous pulmonary valve implantation
PR	pulmonary regurgitation
PS	pulmonary stenosis
PVR	pulmonary vascular resistance
PVRep	pulmonary valve replacement
RA	right atrium
R-L shunt	right-to-left shunt
RPA	right pulmonary artery
RV	right ventricle
RVEF	right ventricular ejection fraction
RVH	right ventricular hypertrophy
RVOT	right ventricular outflow tract
RVOTO	right ventricular outflow tract obstruction
RVP	right ventricular pressure
SCD	sudden cardiac death
SubAS	subaortic stenosis
SupraAS	supravalvular aortic stenosis
SVC	superior vena cava
SVR	systemic vascular resistance
TCPC	total cavopulmonary connection
TEE	transoesophageal echocardiography
TGA	transposition of the great arteries
TGF	transforming growth factor
ToF	tetralogy of Fallot
TR	tricuspid regurgitation

TTE	transthoracic echocardiography
UVH	univentricular heart
VF	ventricular fibrillation
Vmax	maximum Doppler velocity
VSD	ventricular septal defect
VT	ventricular tachycardia
WHO-FC	World Health Organization-functional class
WPW	Wolff-Parkinson-White
WU	Wood units

Introduction

Massimo Chessa and Alessandro Giamberti

The number of people with adult congenital heart disease (ACHD) will inevitably increase in the near future [1]. Recent data suggest that the number of those affected by ACHD, whether repaired or not, approaches the number of children with the disorder [2]. In this growing patient population, Tetralogy of Fallot (ToF) plays a very important role. ToF is the most common form of cyanotic congenital heart disease and thanks to the progress of pediatric cardiac surgery today we can expect that more than 90% of these patients will reach adulthood.

With the increasing number of survivors of surgeries for repair of ToF, the management of possible surgical sequelae, such as chronic pulmonary-valve insufficiency (PVI) and right ventricular (RV) dysfunction, has become a frequent problem. This is a timely topic of increasing clinical interest, as shown by the fact that pulmonary-valve replacement (PVR) for PVI is the operation most frequently reperformed today in ACHD [3, 4]. Long-standing chronic PVI, in these patients, can result in RV dilatation and failure, increasing tricuspid regurgitation, impaired exercise performance, and supraventricular or ventricular arrhythmias. The RV is entirely involved and the pathologies of the RV are becoming more and more frequent. Patients with chronic PVI and RV dysfunction may benefit from earlier reoperations before irreversible myocardial deterioration is established [5–7]. Management of the long-term follow-up of these patients can be difficult and is still under debate. The RV has a more complex anatomy and function than the left ventricle, which makes functional assessment and instrumental evaluation more difficult. The questions of when to reoperate on these patients are becoming increasingly pressing [8]. Clear guidelines to assist in this decision have proved difficult to establish.

M. Chessa (✉)
IRCCS Policlinico San Donato, Pediatric and Adult Congenital Heart Center,
San Donato Milanese (Mi), Italy
e-mail: massichessa@yahoo.it

M. Chessa, A. Giamberti (eds.), *The Right Ventricle in Adults with Tetralogy of Fallot*,
© Springer-Verlag Italia 2012

The percutaneous approach offers a less invasive treatment that may potentially reduce the number of patients for surgery and shift the indications toward earlier intervention. Unfortunately, not all patients are good candidates for transcatheter pulmonary valve implantation because of both the morphology of the RVOT and the residual cardiac anomalies.

Which type of valve to surgically insert into the RVOT is debated. Criteria to take into consideration in this choice should be availability, durability, easy implantation, and facilitation of future interventional procedures.

The research of new devices for surgical and transcatheter approaches will help reduce the number of future reoperations in these patients. At the same time it is undoubtedly clear that stem cell therapies and research in regenerative medicine will dominate the next decade or two, especially directed to the RV.

The management of the RV problems in adult ToF is complex and represents a challenge for the physicians. The objective of this book is to update our knowledge on the assessment, diagnosis and management of all the possible specific problems in a manner that allows physicians to facilitate and plan the management of these patients in their practice.

References

1. Chessa M, Cullen S, Deanfield J et al (2004) The care of adult patient with congenital heart defects: a new challenges. Ital Heart J 5:178-182
2. Webb GD (2001) Care of adults with congenital heart disease. A challenge for the new millennium. J Thorac Cardiovasc Surg 49:30-34
3. Srinathan SK, Bonser RS, Sethia B et al (2004) Changing practice of cardiac surgery in adult patients with congenital heart disease. Heart 91:207-212
4. Giamberti A, Chessa M, Abella R et al (2009) Morbidity and mortality risk factors in adults with congenital heart disease undergoing cardiac reoperation. Ann Thorac Surg 88:1284-1289
5. Therrien J, Siu SC, McLaughlin PR et al (2000) Pulmonary valve replacement in adults late after repair of tetralogy nof Fallot: are we operating too late? J Am Coll Cardiol 36:1670-1675
6. Frigiola A, Tsang V, Bull C et al (2008) Biventricular response following pulmonary valve replacement for right ventricular outflow tract dysfunction. Is age predictor of outcome? Circulation 118(14 suppl):S182-190
7. Frigiola A, Giamberti A, Chessa M et al (2006) Right ventricular restoration during pulmonary valve implantation in adults with congenital heart disease. Eur J Cardiothorac Surg 29(suppl):S279-85
8. Harrild DM, Berul CI, Cecchin F et al (2009) Pulmonary valve replacement in tetralogy of Fallot. Impact on survival and ventricular tachycardia. Circulation 119:445-451

Anatomy of Tetralogy of Fallot

Carla Frescura and Gaetano Thiene

2.1 History

It was Etienne-Louis Arthur Fallot who, in 1888, first described the clinico-pathological correlates of the "maladie bleue" [1]. The lesion that he identified was the association of interventricular communication, sub pulmonary stenosis, biventricular origin of the aorta and hypertrophy of the right ventricle. From the translation in English by Allwork in 1988 [2], come the following significant passages of Fallot's original work:

> … during the last few years, three cases of a rare and curious disease have passed before our eyes…observed during their lives and afterwards at necropsy, three patients affected by the illness called "maladie bleue".
> …we thought that the "maladie bleue" was caused by these lesions multiple but constant, so together they constituted a type perfectly defined.
> All the three patients had… an abnormal interventricular communication and in each of them the ventricular septal defect was in the same place, the superior part of the septum…the pulmonary artery was narrowed and in each there was subarterial as well as valvular stenosis…there was ventricular hypertrophy…the aorta deviated to the right…took equal origin from both ventricles."

Nowadays it is well known that this combination of anomalies had been recognized long before Fallot's description [3]. In retrospect, some examples of this malformation had been illustrated by Stenonis (1671–1672) [4], Farre (1814) [5], Peacock (1866) [6] and Von Rokitansky (1875) [7]. Stenonis had described the findings in a fetus with bifid sternum and omphalocele, syn-

G. Thiene (✉)
Department of Cardiological, Thoracic and Vascular Sciences, University of Padua,
Padua, Italy
e-mail: gaetano.thiene@unipd.it

M. Chessa, A. Giamberti (eds.), *The Right Ventricle in Adults with Tetralogy of Fallot*,
© Springer-Verlag Italia 2012

dactyly and cleft palate, first reporting the frequent presence of associated extra cardiac malformations [4]. The merit of Fallot was to correlate the pathological findings with the clinical features.

It was Maude Abbott who coined the name "Tetralogy of Fallot" (ToF) in 1924 [8], believing this designation more convenient than the simple list of the four cardiac anomalies [9].

Even within the morphological definition, no two hearts with ToF are identical [10, 11]. The variation in phenotypic framework includes the difference in the margin of the interventricular communication, the extent of aortic overriding and the degree of pulmonary obstruction.

The fourth component of tetralogy, the right ventricular hypertrophy, is the hemodynamic consequence of the associated malformations with a systemic right ventricle.

From the anatomic point of view, ToF represents a morphological spectrum with at one end, hearts with ventricular septal defect (VSD) and aortic overriding with minimal pulmonary stenosis, and at the other end, hearts with ventricular septal defect, aortic overriding and pulmonary atresia.

2.2   Normal Anatomy of Right Ventricular Outflow

Different from the left ventricular outflow tract, which is wedged in between the inflow of the atrioventricular (AV) valves and strictly related to the mitral valve (mitro-aortic fibrous continuity), the right ventricular outflow tract is anteriorly located, far from the tricuspid valve and from the inflow of the right ventricle (Fig. 2.1).

The topography of the right ventricular outflow tract is delineated by discrete muscular structures. Proximally it starts from the moderator band, which connects the anterior papillary muscle of the tricuspid valve to the trabecula septomarginalis (TSM), a distinct muscular structure located on the right side and reinforcing the ventricular septum. Distally, the TSM bifurcates like a sling into two limbs, one anterior, joining the pulmonary valve, and one posterior, lying over the membranous septum. This sling accommodates the so-called crista supraventricularis, which goes from the septal to the lateral free wall. The musculature of the inner curvature of the heart (ventriculo infundibular fold) constitutes the greater part of this structure. The lateral part of the crista separates the anterior leaflet of the tricuspid valve from the pulmonary valve (tricuspid-pulmonary muscular discontinuity) and the septal part represents the so-called infundibular/outlet septum.

By definition, the outlet septum is the muscular structure that, within the ventricular cavity, separates the subaortic from the subpulmonary outlets. In the normal heart there is virtually no, or a very small, muscular septum interposed between the ventricular outlets, because the pulmonary valve is lifted away from the base of the ventricle. In this way the so-called outlet septum separates the pulmonary infundibulum from the right aortic cusp rather than

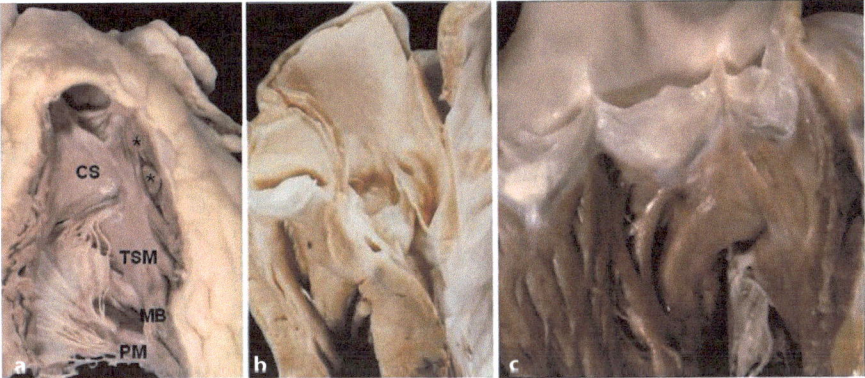

Fig. 2.1 Anatomy of the right ventricular outflow. **a** In the right ventricular outflow a prominent muscular structure, the trabecula septo marginalis (*TSM*), is present. In the proximal part it is connected with the moderator band (*MB*) and the anterior papillary muscle (*PM*) of the tricuspid valve. On the distal end it bifurcates into two limbs that delimitate the crista supraventricularis (*CS*) that separates the pulmonary and tricuspid valves. Note the presence of the septo-parietal bands (***). **b** View of the right and left ventricular outflows: note the higher position of the pulmonary valve, due to the presence of the crista supraventricularis, and the lower position of the aortic valve as a consequence of the fibrous continuity with the mitral valve. Only a small part of the outlet septum separates the right from the left ventricle, while a large part separates the pulmonary infundibulum from the aortic sinusal tract. **c** The pulmonary valve is separated from the tricuspid valve by interposition of a muscular structure (crista supraventricularis) and all the three cusps are attached to the myocardium

from the left ventricular outflow tract. During resection of the infundibular septum, the risk of entering into the aorta must be considered.

In the pulmonary infundibulum other muscular structures with prominent intertrabecular spaces are usually present: namely the septo-parietal bands that arise from the septum and join the anterior wall of the right ventricular outflow tract.

The end of the right ventricular outflow is marked by the pulmonary valve, which consists of three semilunar cusps (one anterior and two posterior, right and left) facing the corresponding aortic left and right anterior cusps. The base of all the pulmonary cusps is attached to the myocardium of the right ventricular outflow tract, which, different from the left ventricular outflow tract, is entirely represented by cardiac muscle.

The medial papillary muscle of the tricuspid valve (also known as conal or Lancisi's papillary muscle) is situated at the bifurcation (sling) of the TSM and is the landmark of the right bundle branch in its septal course. The right bundle branch turns down at this level, to run into the subendocardium of the TSM and, after a division, part of the right bundle branch courses in the moderator band and reaches the anterior papillary muscle of the tricuspid valve.

2.3   Anatomy of Tetralogy of Fallot

2.3.1   Pulmonary Stenosis

Although ToF can be diagnosed by the contemporary presence of the four cardiac defects, the landmark of this anomaly is the abnormal antero-cephalad deviation of the outlet septum, malaligned with respect to the rest of the muscular ventricular septum [12–15]. If in the normal heart the outlet septum is a poorly developed structure, on the contrary in ToF the outlet septum is an extensive right ventricular structure that has no counterpart in the normal heart. The deviation of the outlet septum is per se responsible for the coexistence of the narrowed subpulmonary infundibulum, of the large subaortic VSD and of the biventricular origin of the aorta (Fig. 2.2). The deviation of the outlet septum associated with subaortic VSD and overriding aorta can be found also in the absence of subpulmonary obstruction as in the Eisenmenger complex [16, 17]. In ToF the narrowing of the subpulmonary infundibulum is due both to the deviated outlet septum and abnormal morphology of the septo-parietal bands, which reinforces the parietal wall of the right ventricle (Fig. 2.3) [18–21]. The septo-parietal bands are muscular structures, also present in the

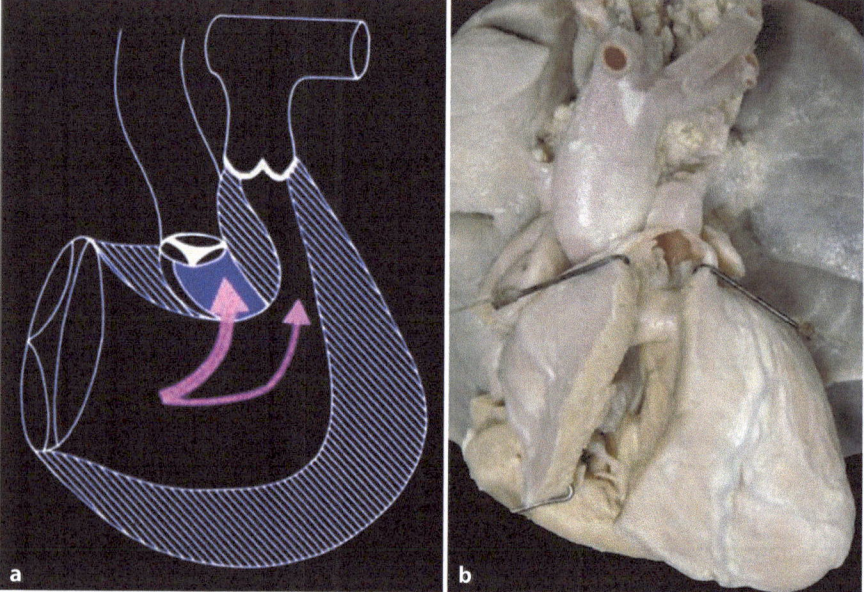

Fig. 2.2 a Schematic representation of the malformation characterized by valvular and subvalvular pulmonary stenosis, ventricular septal defect, overriding aorta and right ventricular hypertrophy. **b** Anatomical specimen with subpulmonary stenosis due to deviation of the outlet septum and stenotic and dysplastic pulmonary valve

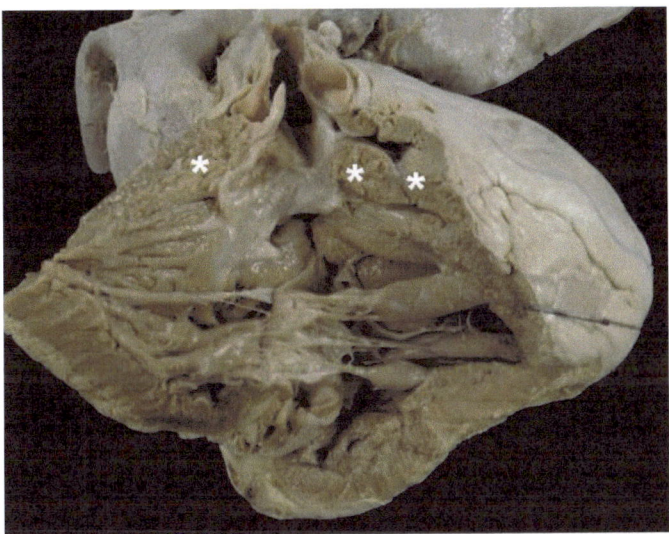

Fig. 2.3 View of the right ventricular outflow: the subpulmonary stenosis is due to deviation of the outlet septum and severe hypertrophy of the septo-parietal bands (*). A dysplastic and stenotic pulmonary valve is also present

normal heart, which extend from the TSM to the free wall of the pulmonary infundibulum. In hearts with ToF the septo-parietal bands are abnormally hypertrophied, contributing to subpulmonary obstruction.

Van Praagh et al. [21, 22] asserted that the basic anatomy of ToF is the consequence of the "underdevelopment of the sub pulmonary infundibulum that appears too small, too short, too narrow and too shallow".

Whilst the subpulmonary infundibulum results narrowed, subsequent anatomical [12, 23, 24] and echocardiographic studies [25] have shown that it is significantly longer than in the normal heart and that the malaligned outlet septum in ToF is a much more prominent structure than the one found in the normal outflow of the heart [25]. Only occasionally hearts exhibit a hypoplastic and short subpulmonary infundibulum, particularly in ToF with pulmonary atresia. In the majority of hearts the muscular outlet septum is much more prominent than in normal hearts and often hypertrophied.

The degree of deviation of the outlet septum also affects the growth of the pulmonary arteries: a linear correlation exists with the degree of obstruction and the development of the pulmonary arterial tree. Pulmonary valvular stenosis is a frequent accompaniment [25]. The valve can show three stenotic cusps (Fig. 2.4a), or a unicommissural dome shape aspect (Fig. 2.4c). More frequently the stenotic valve is bicuspid and dysplastic (Fig. 2.4b) [15]. The valvular lesion is rarely the major cause of obstruction.

Further narrowing of the subpulmonary infundibulum is often due to superimposed accretions of fibrous tissue on the endocardium.

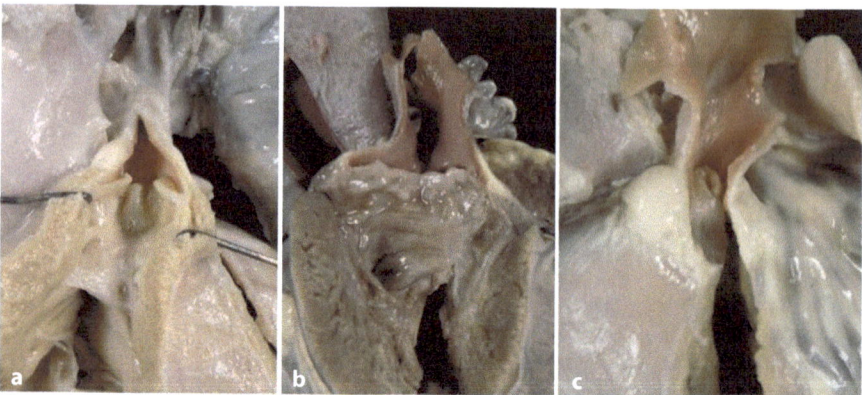

Fig. 2.4 The pulmonary valvular stenosis can coexist with the deviation of the outlet septum. **a** Tricuspid and dysplastic valve. **b** Bicuspid and dysplastic valve. **c** Unicuspid valve

2.3.2 Ventricular Septal Defect

The VSD is the consequence of the deviation of the outlet septum or of its fibrous remnant that fail to muscularize during the embryologic development [19, 20, 26]. The VSD is subaortic, located in the basal portion of the ventricular septum and associated with malaligment between the outlet septum itself and the remainder of the interventricular septum. The size can vary but usually the VSD is of large dimensions.

The most frequent type (nearly 80% of cases) is the perimembranous defect characterized by fibrous continuity between the tricuspid, mitral and aortic valve in its postero-inferior rim (Fig. 2.5a). This defect involves the membranous septum in part or totally, and extends into the muscular septum. The AV conduction axis runs in the postero-inferior rim of the defect and it is at risk of injury during patch closure of the VSD [27, 28].

In the muscular type (about 20% of cases) all the borders are muscular and there is no fibrous continuity between the aorta and the tricuspid valve at the postero-inferior rim of the defect (Fig. 2.5b). The presence of this muscular structure protects the His bundle during the closure of the defect [27, 28].

The third type of defect is characterized by the presence of an antero superior rim made up of a fibrous raphe between the cusps of the aortic and pulmonary valves (Fig. 2.5c). This type of defect is rare in Caucasians but seems to be more frequent in Central and South America and the Far East. In this case the outlet septum failed to develop and the defect can be classified as subarterial or doubly committed, because of its location both in the subpulmonary and subaortic position [26]. This type of defect can be defined as perimembranous or muscular according to the morphology of its poster-inferior rim. In the past some authors have argued that, since the outlet septum was not present in this defect, a ToF cannot be recognized [14, 15, 29]. Actually, a

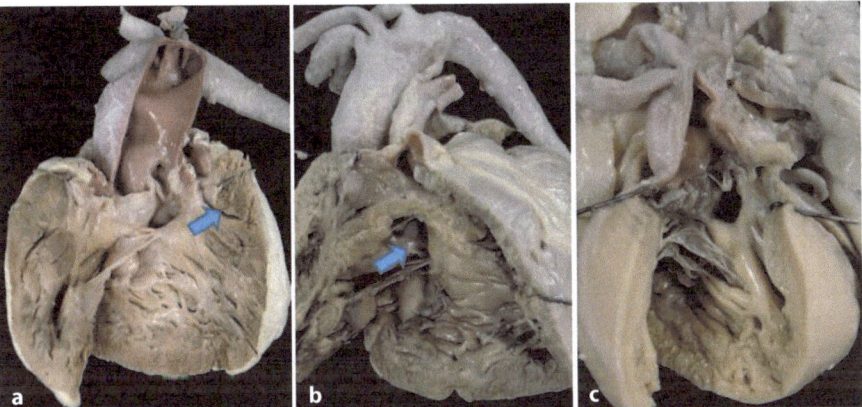

Fig. 2.5 a View from the right ventricle: note the extreme hypoplasia of the subpulmonary infundibulum (*arrow*), the overriding aorta and the large perimembranous ventricular septal defect. A fibrous continuity between the aortic valve and the tricuspid valve is present at the postero-inferior rim of the defect. **b** In this specimen, viewed from the right ventricle, a muscular infundibular ventricular defect is present (*arrow*), surrounded by a muscular rim. Note the hypoplastic pulmonary artery and the infundibular stenosis due to the deviated outlet septum. **c** In this case the outlet septum is absent and the ventricular defect is subarterial. Note the fibrous postero-inferior rim of the defect (perimembranous defect)

remnant of the outlet septum seems to be present as a malaligned fibrous raphe beneath the conjoined cusps of the arterial valves, causing obstruction of the right outflow [19, 20, 26].

The VSD can also extend into the inlet component of the ventricle in the presence of an AV septal defect or in association with malaligment between the atria and the ventricular septal structures with straddling or overriding tricuspid valve.

2.3.3 Aortic Override

In the normal heart the aortic valve cusps are attached exclusively within the left ventricle and a fibrous continuity exists between the anterior mitral leaflet and the left coronary and posterior non coronary aortic cusps. When the subaortic ventricular septum is deficient, part of the aortic valve circumference can be supported by the right ventricular structures (Figs. 2.5, 2.6). This aortic overriding is obviously accentuated in the presence of deviation of the outlet septum as in ToF and in Eisenmenger complex [16, 17]. The degree of override can vary and, when the aorta is supported predominantly by the left ventricle (more than 50%) the ventriculo-arterial connection is concordant. If the aorta is predominantly supported by the right ventricle (more than 50%), a double outlet ventricular connection is present. That is not in contrast with the

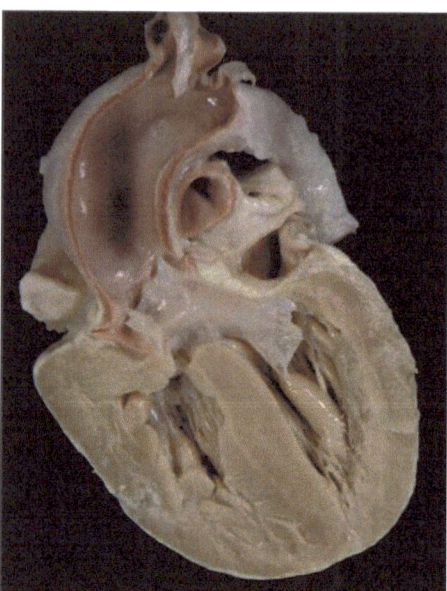

Fig. 2.6 Anatomic section in long axis of a specimen with ToF showing the aortic overriding and a perimembranous ventricular septal defect

definition of tetralogy because in this case the double outlet right ventricle is considered as a type of ventriculo-arterial connection [18–20]. The anatomical entity of double outlet right ventricle with subaortic VSD is characterized by the origin of both the semilunar valve predominantly from the right ventricle associated with bilateral muscular infundibulum and absence of mitro-aortic continuity.

2.3.4 Associated Anomalies

Several cardiac lesions can be associated with ToF.

The most severe is the association with pulmonary atresia [30–33], the extreme form of pulmonary obstruction. In this condition the lungs can be supplied by a patent ductus arteriosus or by collateral systemic-to-pulmonary arteries originating from the aorta (Fig. 2.7). The presence of large collateral arteries can be responsible for left-to-right shunt and the early onset of a hypertensive pulmonary vascular disease [31].

An AV septal defect is found in 13% of cases with ToF [34–36], rendering the surgical repair more complex. A common AV valve is the rule, but rare cases are reported with two separated AV valves (the so-called intermediate type of AV septal defect) [35]. In nearly all patients the superior common leaflet is free floating, corresponding to type C morphology of Rastelli classification (Fig. 2.8). Usually the common valve is competent, however there are

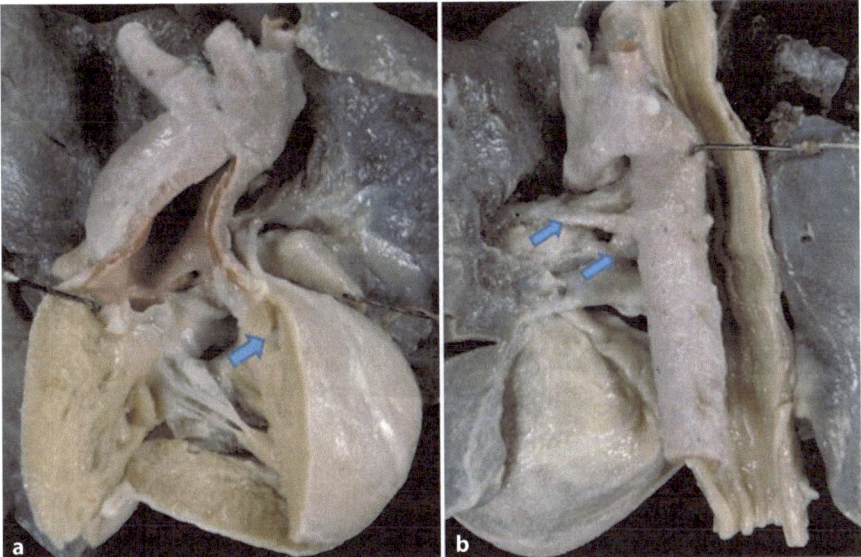

Fig. 2.7 ToF with pulmonary atresia and systemic collateral circulation. **a** Right ventricular outflow: a blind infundibulum (*arrow*) is present and the aorta overrides a perimembranous ventricular septal defect. Note the diminutive pulmonary artery. **b** Posterior view of the same specimen: multiple collateral systemic-to-pulmonary arteries take origin from the descending aorta and supply the lungs (*arrows*)

cases with dysplastic leaflets. ToF in association with AV septal defect occurs characteristically, but not exclusively, in patients with Down syndrome.

A patent foramen ovale or an ostium secundum atrial septal defect are frequently observed and additional muscular septal defects can be noted (Fig. 2.8). The presence of an interatrial septal defect was reported by Fallot himself [1] and the situation is known as pentalogy of Fallot.

Anomalies of the mitral valve such as cleft of the anterior leaflet, double orifice or parachute mitral valve (Fig. 2.9) have been also reported.

Straddling or overriding tricuspid valves may also occur, complicating the closure of the interventricular defect.

Accessory atrioventricular tissue can be found due to the presence of a fibrous flap representing a remnant of the membranous septum or of accessory tissue related to the tricuspid valve [37, 38]. A perimembranous VSD is regularly associated in these cases. We have described two types of these accessory tags: a mobile type obstructing the interventricular defect and ballooning into the subaortic region potentially obstructing the left outflow tract, and a fixed type, strictly anchored by chordae tendineae to the interventricular septum [37]. Sometimes this accessory tissue can be used for the anchorage of the interventricular patch, avoiding damaging the conduction tissue running on the infero-posterior rim of the perimembranous defect [39].

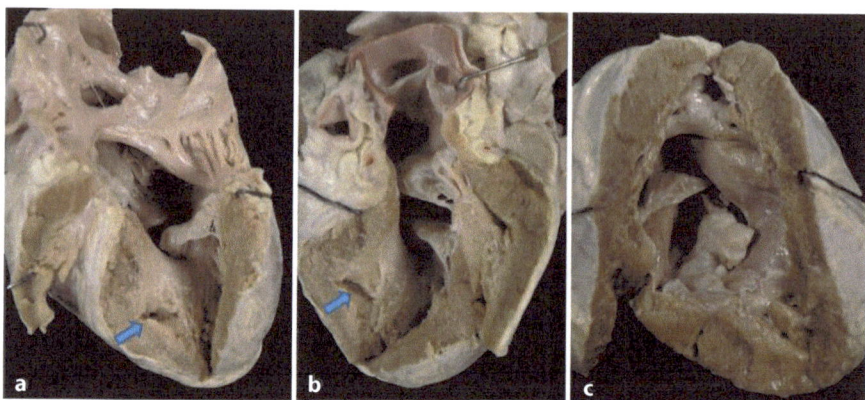

Fig. 2.8 ToF with AV septal defect. **a** View from the left cardiac chambers: a large AV septal defect is present with a common AV valve. Note the presence of an additional interatrial septal defect, fossa ovalis type, and of a muscular ventricular septal defect in the trabecular portion of the ventricular septum (*arrow*). **b** View of the left outflow tract: the common AV valve shows a free floating superior leaflet without chordal insertion to the crest of the ventricular septum (AV septal defect type C of Rastelli classification). Note the overriding position of the aorta. The *arrow* indicates the additional muscular VSD. **c** Outlet of the right ventricle with severe infundibular stenosis due to the deviated outlet septum and endocardial plaques

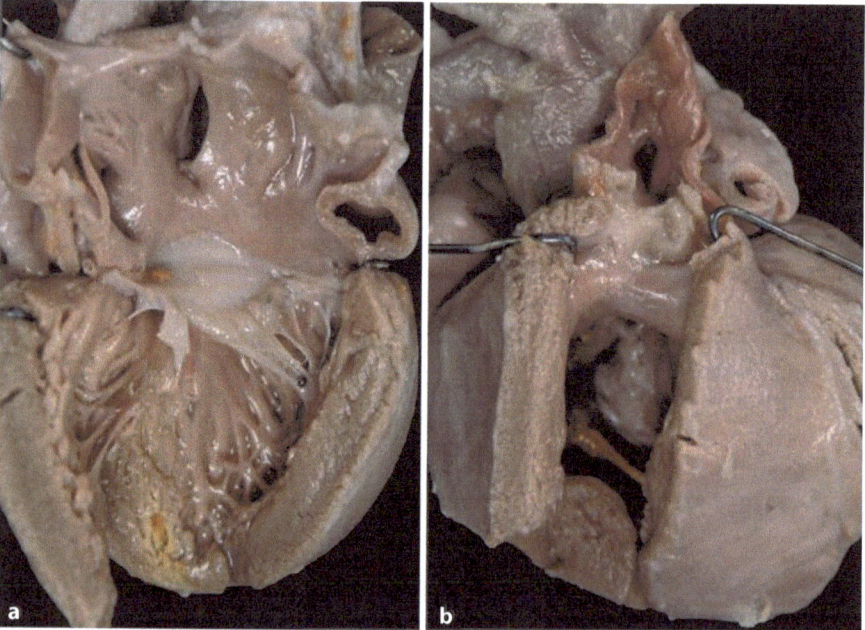

Fig. 2.9 ToF with mitral valve anomaly. **a** View from the left cardiac chambers: most of the chordae tendineae of the mitral leaflets are attached to the anterior papillary muscle mimicking parachute morphology. **b** View from the subpulmonary infundibulum: note the deviated outlet septum and the dysplastic and stenotic pulmonary valve

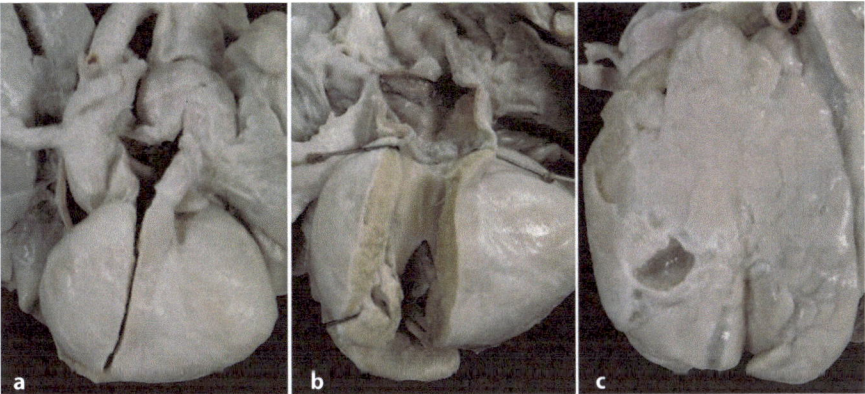

Fig. 2.10 ToF with absent pulmonary valve. **a** External view of the heart: an aneurysmatic left pulmonary artery compresses the left bronchus. **b** View of the right outflow: note the subpulmonary stenosis due to deviated outlet septum, which is the landmark of ToF. The pulmonary cusps are almost absent with fibrous-myxoid nodular remnants. The pulmonary annulus is stenotic and the common pulmonary trunk is dilated. **c** The lung shows emphysema due to entrapping of the air by bronchial compression

The arterial duct can be present (patent or closed) or absent.

The ductus is usually absent in association with the so-called absence of the pulmonary valve [40–42]. In these cases the pulmonary cusps are substituted by annular fibrous rudiments (Fig. 2.10) resulting in pulmonary regurgitation also during fetal life. The pulmonary artery, trunk and/or branches can be markedly dilated causing compression of the bronchi (Fig. 2.10).

A right aortic arch with a mirror image branching of the brachiocephalic arteries (Fig. 2.11) is observed in 50% of cases of ToF. An aberrant origin of the left subclavian artery is not uncommon in this setting [43] and a vascular ring can be found in the presence of a patent ductus or ligamentum arteriosus (Fig. 2.12) [28]. Also a double aortic arch can be found (Fig. 2.13). In the presence of these vascular rings, respiratory distress and/or dysphagia can be related to compression of trachea or esophagus respectively. Also a retro esophageal course of the right subclavian artery in the left aortic arch may be present in the absence of obstruction of trachea and esophagus (Fig. 2.14).

Dilatation of the aortic root is a clinical feature present in unrepaired ToF but also in patients after surgery (Fig. 2.11). In some cases aortic regurgitation may occur, requiring aortic valve replacement and rarely the dilated ascending aorta is at risk of rupture or dissection. Histological abnormalities, such as cystic medial necrosis, fibrosis and disruption of the elastic lamellae are observed in patients from an early age, suggesting the presence of an intrinsic pathology of the aortic wall from birth [44]. The exact mechanism (hemodynamic stress, genes, etc.) for the underlying histological abnormalities is unclear.

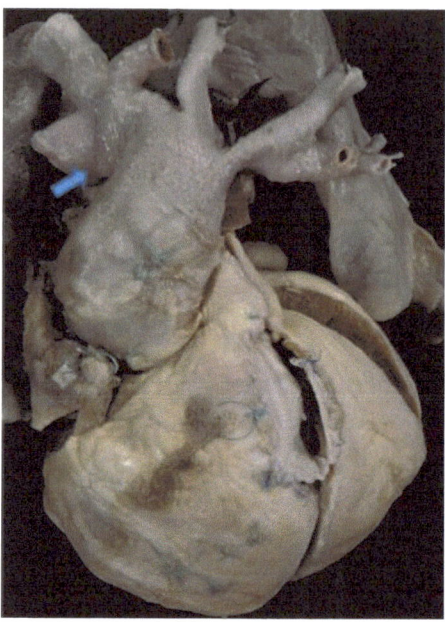

Fig. 2.11 ToF and right aortic arch. External view of the heart in a patient who underwent surgical repair. The specimen shows a right aortic arch with mirror image origin of the brachiocefalic arteries. The *arrow* indicates the descending aorta in the right aortic arch. Note the dilated ascending aorta

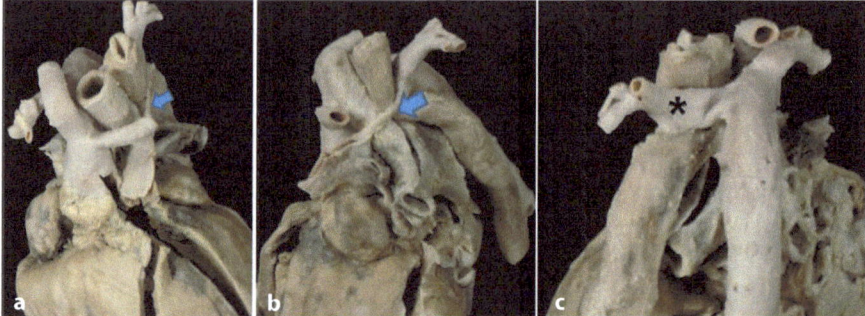

Fig. 2.12 ToF with vascular ring. **a** External view of the heart. A vascular ring is present due to right aortic arch, retro esophageal left subclavian artery and left ligamentum arteriosus (*arrow*). The ring encircles the trachea and the esophagus. **b** Lateral view: the left ligamentum arteriosus (*arrow*), connecting the pulmonary artery with the left subclavian artery, is responsible for compression of trachea and strangulation of esophagus accounting for dysphagia. **c** Posterior view: note the right descending aorta and the retroesophageal left subclavian artery (*)

Stenosis of the pulmonary arteries, usually located at the branching site, are also an important associated malformation for their surgical significance. Lack of origin of a pulmonary artery, usually the left one, is not infrequent and the corresponding lung is supplied by a patent ductus arteriosus. Origin of a pulmonary artery directly from the ascending aorta has been also reported.

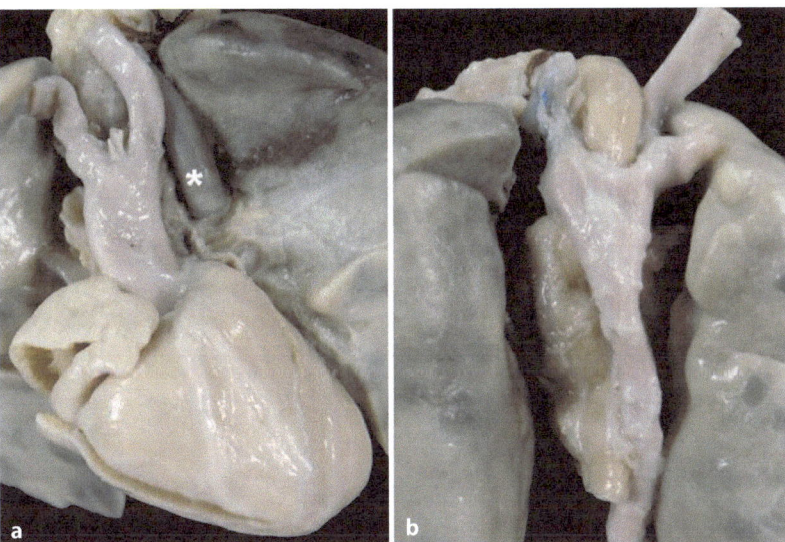

Fig. 2.13 ToF with double aortic arch. **a** Anterior view of the heart: note the hypoplastic pulmonary artery and the presence of a surgical shunt (*) between the left subclavian artery and the left pulmonary artery. **b** Posterior view of the heart showing the two aortic arches, both patent, merging into a single descending aorta

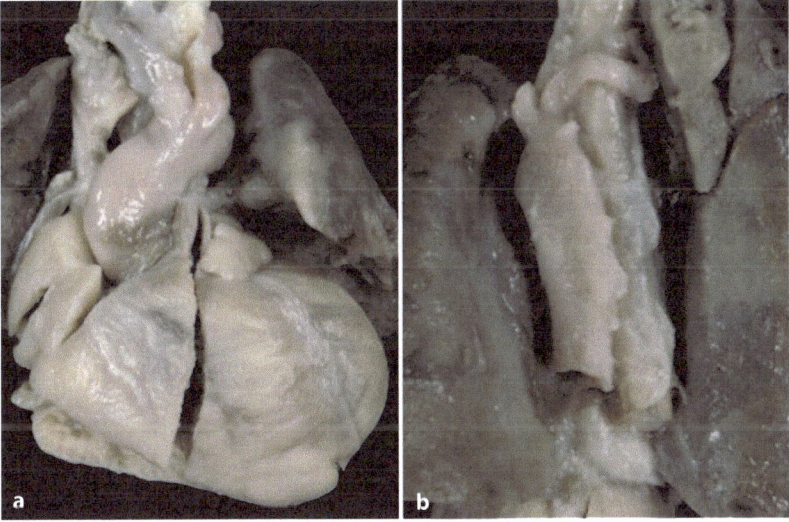

Fig. 2.14 ToF with retro esophageal right subclavian artery. **a** Anterior view of the heart with hypoplastic pulmonary trunk dilated aorta and left aortic arch. **b** Posterior view of the same specimen. The descending aorta is on the left side. The right subclavian artery takes origin from the left aortic arch and runs behind the esophagus (retroesophageal right subclavian artery)

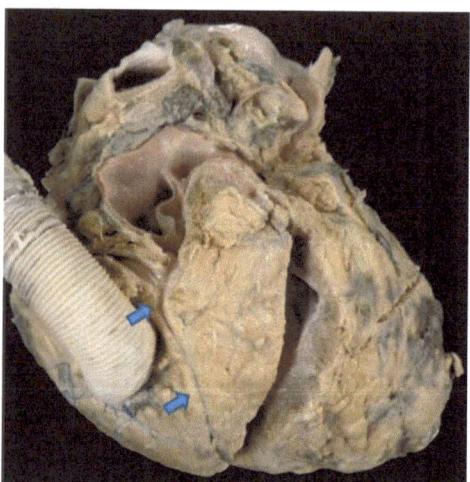

Fig. 2.15 ToF with coronary artery anomaly. In this patient a valved conduit was used to reconstruct the right ventricle-to-pulmonary artery continuity, to avoid infundibulotomy as a consequence of a coronary artery anomaly, unrecognized preoperatively. A large conal artery (*arrows*) originates from the right coronary artery and runs parallel to the descending anterior coronary artery

Sometimes collateral systemic-to-pulmonary arteries can be associated with ToF and pulmonary stenosis, even if they are usually observed in the setting of pulmonary atresia.

Two chambered right ventricles can occur due to hypertrophy of the apical portion of the trabecula septomarginalis or of the moderator band.

The coronary arteries can show anomalies of origin and course. The incidence of a major coronary artery crossing the right ventricular outflow occurs in between 5 and 12% of cases. The most significant malformation is the origin of the anterior descending coronary artery from the right coronary artery and its course across the anterior subepicardial surface of the pulmonary infundibulum. In some cases a high take off of the right or left coronary artery was reported [45] with an origin above the sino tubular junction and intramural course in the aortic wall. This fact may be responsible for sudden death, especially during exercise. Accessory coronary ostia (one or two) can be observed in the right aortic sinus giving origin to one or more conal branches [45]. These branches do not represent a contraindication to ventriculotomy in the correction of ToF, unless they are equal in caliber or larger than the right coronary artery. It is only the aberrant anterior descending coronary artery or any other artery arising from the right coronary artery and crossing the outflow tract which is a serious risk if unrecognized during ventriculotomy (Fig. 2.15).

ToF may be also associated with extra cardiac anomalies and genetic syndromes. Associated chromosomal anomalies can include trisomies 21, 18 and 13. Recent studies emphasized that ToF is frequently associated with branchial arch defects including Di George syndrome, velocardiofacial and conotruncal anomaly and face syndromes with microdeletion of chromosome 22q11 (CATCH 22) [46, 47]. In these patients a frequent presence of subarterial VSD and right aortic arch was noted [46].

2.4   Postoperative Pathology

The steps for ToF repair are the closure of the VSD and the relief of the right ventricular outflow tract obstruction, which may be localized at subvalvular, valvular and supravalvular pulmonary levels. According to Kirklin [48], the optimal result is achieved when the postoperative RV/LV systemic pressure ratio is less than 0,5.

Resection of myocardium in the free wall of the pulmonary infundibulum, including septo-parietal bands, is an intrinsic part of the operation and may be accomplished through an atrial approach. The relief of septo-marginal bands, where the right bundle branch is localized, may be the cause of postoperative right bundle branch block.

The deviated infundibular septum is usually spared from resection, because of the risk of damage to the aortic cusp attachment on the opposite left side.

In the majority of cases the obstruction is also a consequence of hypoplasia of the pulmonary annulus and of the pulmonary artery. This obstacle can be relieved with a transanular pericardial patch, either autologous or glutaraldehyde fixed xenograft. This implies infundibulotomy for insertion of the proximal patch, a procedure at risk of myocardial infarction if it damages the conal arteries or the anterior descending coronary artery when originating abnormally from the right coronary artery (Fig. 2.15) [28]. Knowledge of coronary artery anatomy patterns through preoperative coronary arteriography is essential before infundibulotomy [45]. The transvalvular patch should include a valve apparatus (usually a homograft or xenograft semilunar cusp) in order to prevent postoperative pulmonary regurgitation. In the long term, calcification of both patch and cusp may occur, with pulmonary stenosis or incompetence. Pulmonary incompetence or stenosis may be nowadays managed without thoracotomy by transcatheter valve implantation [49].

Distal obstruction because of pulmonary artery hypoplasia at bifurcation requires a precise preoperative angiographic visualization, otherwise a significant residual stenosis may be expected. Focal stenosis may occur following previous Blalock Taussig shunt, at the site of the pulmonary anastomosis. This is one of the reasons why one stage early total repair is currently recommended.

The complications of the closure of the VSD, nowadays accomplished through atrial approach but once closed through infudibulotomy approach, may consist of patch dehiscence (Fig. 2.16) and injury of the AV conducting tissues (Fig. 2.17) [28]. This was a frequent complication in the early days of cardiac surgery, when the disposition of the AV conduction axis was still unknown to the surgeon. The early experience of Kirklin at the Mayo Clinic in the operation of VSD resulted in 50% postoperative AV block [50]. The risk is particularly high in perimembranous VSD, where the His bundle with bifurcation is bare at the postero-inferior rim of the defect (Fig. 2.17) [27, 28]. By suturing the patch, the His bundle may be transected or involved by hemorrhage. Postoperative AV block with permanent pace-maker implantation is

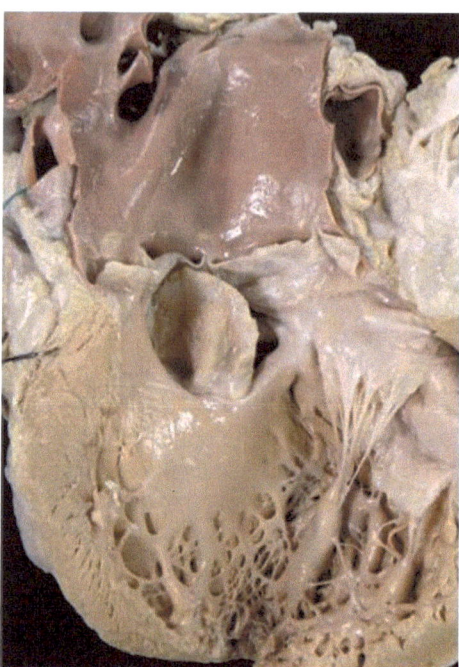

Fig. 2.16 Postoperative ToF. Partial detachment of the interventricular patch interferes with the normal function of the aortic valve. Note the dilatation of the left ventricle due to aortic incompetence

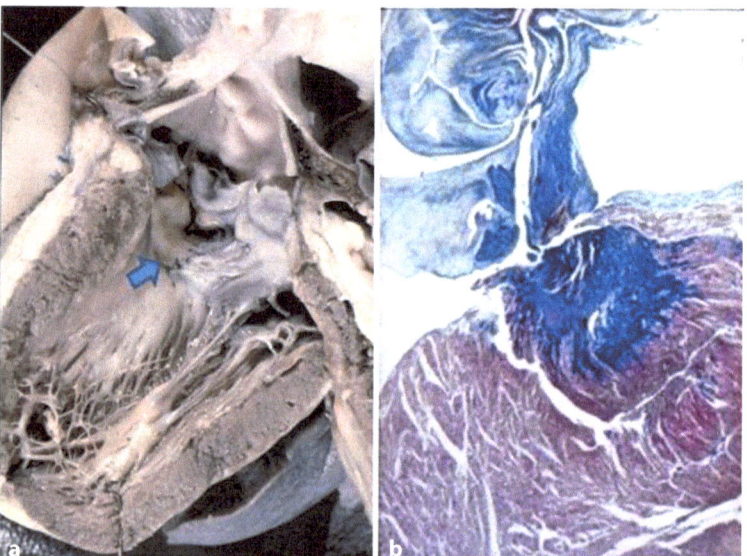

Fig. 2.17 Postoperative ToF. **a** Left view of the interventricular septum in a patient who died of AV block after surgical repair. The *arrow* indicates surgical sutures at the postero-inferior rim of the perimembranous ventricular septal defect. **b** Histological section of the same area showing the traumatic disruption of the branching bundle by suture (Azan stain, original magnification x8)

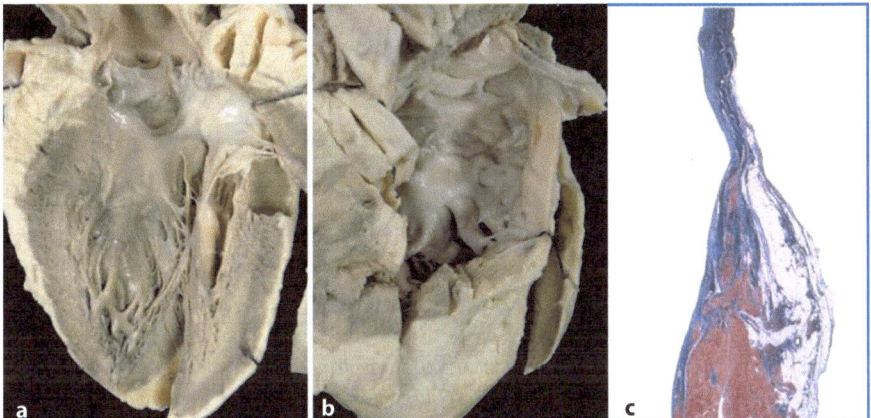

Fig. 2.18 Postoperative ToF. Sudden death in a patient operated upon by transannular patch. **a** View from the left ventricle: note the patch used for the closure of the perimembranous ventricular septal defect inserted far from the postero-inferior rim without damage of the His bundle. **b** View from the right outflow: the pulmonary stenosis was relieved by transannular patch and the right infundibulum is severely dilated. **c** The histology of the pulmonary infundibulum shows the patch with the scarry of the right ventricular myocardium (Azan stain, original magnification x5)

nowadays quite rare, since the surgeon is well aware of the disposition of the conduction system, anchoring the patch on tricuspid valve tissue at the postero-inferior rim in the presence of perimembranous VSD.

In case of severe stenosis or atresia of the pulmonary outflow tract, the obstruction may be relieved through a valved conduit from the right ventricle to the pulmonary artery (if large enough in size), thus restoring right ventricle-pulmonary artery continuity. Several conduits have been employed (aortic porcine, aortic or pulmonary valve homograft, bovine jugular vein, bovine pericardium), all with disappointing results because of late complications like fibrous pannus or calcification as well as the occurrence of mismatch with the growth of the child.

In cases of pulmonary atresia, with pulmonary circulation supported by collateral systemic to pulmonary arteries, the aim of surgery is the unifocalization of the arterial supply so that the entire pulmonary arterial circulation is connected with the restored right ventricle-pulmonary artery continuity [51–53]. If the arterial lung perfusion (lobe or segments) has been supported for a long time by systemic, non obstructed, collateral arteries, focal or diffuse pulmonary vascular disease may have developed, with severe pulmonary hypertension after total repair [31].

Finally, a sword of Damocles is hanging, although with rare occurrence, in repaired ToF. We refer to sudden arrhythmic death due to ventricular fibrillation. The fibrous scar around the infudibulotomy/infudibulectomy may threaten the electrical stability of the right ventricle, which is transformed in arrhythmogenic right ventricular disease (Fig. 2.18) [54]. Right ventricular dilatation due to pulmonary valve incompetence and poor ejection fracture due to excessive infundibular muscle resection may aggravate the electrically instability, as to require implantable defibrillator.

2.5   Anatomical Collection of the University of Padua

In the Anatomical Collection of the University of Padua, of among 1,543 hearts with congenital heart disease collected from 1968 to 2011, 123 hearts were affected by ToF (7.9%) (pulmonary atresia excluded).

ToF was isolated in 95 (77%) cases, associated with AV septal defect in 17 (14%) and with absent pulmonary valve cusps in 11 (9%).

The age ranged from 0 days to 55 years. The median age of death was 4 years in isolated forms, 7 month in cases with AV septal defect and 10 days in cases with absent pulmonary cusps.

52 patients were female and 71 male. 13 were fetal hearts. 19 patients underwent palliative surgery, 60 to complete surgical repair and four to heart transplantation. Three patients died suddenly, all far from surgical repair.

The associated cardiac and extracardiac anomalies in the different groups are summarized in Tables 2.1 and 2.2.

The perimembranous outlet defect was the most frequent VSD with an incidence of 80% (Fig. 2.5a). The muscular VSD accounted for about the 20% of cases (Fig. 2.5b) and the sub arterial defects were quite rare (Fig. 2.5c).

There was a high incidence of right aortic arch (17%) (Fig. 2.11) and bicuspid pulmonary valve (Fig. 2.4b). The pulmonary valve was rarely unicuspid (Fig. 2.4c).

The left pulmonary artery was absent in one case and in one other case a pulmonary sling was present with the left branch running between esophagus and trachea.

In two cases a vascular ring was present consisting of a double aortic arch in one (Fig. 2.13) and a right aortic arch, retro esophageal subclavian artery and left ligamentum arteriosus in the other (Fig. 2.12).

In three patients (aged 2, 4 and 43 years) collateral systemic/to-pulmonary arteries were noted.

The anomalies of the mitral (cleft, parachute [Fig. 2.9], double orifice) or tricuspid valves were rare. Accessory AV tissue was found in four cases, fixed in two and mobile in the others.

In ToF with AV septal defect the anterior leaflet of the common valve was free floating (AV septal type C of Rastelli classification) in all (Fig. 2.8) and the incidence of trisomy 21 was higher than in isolated form (36% versus 6%).

Patients with ToF and absent pulmonary cusps (Fig. 2.10) presented less associated malformations and in our series no chromosomal anomalies. In this group of hearts, agenesis of the ductus arteriosus was noted in all cases except the one with absent left pulmonary artery where the ductus arteriosus supplied the left lung.

Table 2.1 Associated cardiac anomalies in ToF in the Anatomical Collection of the University of Padua (123 cases)

Anomalies	Isolated ToF 95 hearts (77%)	ToF + AV septal defect 17 hearts (14%)	ToF + absent pulmonary valve 11 hearts (9%)	Total 123 hearts
Perimembranous outlet VSD	73 (77%)	-	8 (73%)	**81 (76%)**
Perimembranous inlet VSD	1*	-	-	1*
Muscular outlet VSD	20 (21%)	-	2 (18%)	**22 (20%)**
Muscular trabecular VSD	-	1*	-	1*
Sub arterial VSD	2	-	1	3
Persistent left SVC	7	4	-	11
Absent coronary sinus	-	2	-	2
Tricuspid double orifice	1	-	-	1
Accessory AV tissue	4	-	-	4
Mitral double orifice	1	-	-	1
Mitral cleft	2	-	-	2
Parachute mitral valve	2	-	-	2
Unicuspid pulmonary valve	5	1	-	6
Bicuspid pulmonary valve	33 (35%)	2 (11%)	-	**35 (28%)**
Absent left pulmonary branch	-	-	1	1
Pulmonary sling	1	-	-	1
Bicuspid aortic valve	1	1	-	2
Aortic valve prolapse	4	-	-	4
Coronary anomalies	4	-	-	4
Right aortic arch	16 (17%)	3 (17%)	2 (18%)	**21 (17%)**
Double aortic arch	1	-	-	1
Vascular ring	1	-	-	1
Retro esophageal right subclavian artery	4	2	1	7
Absent ductus	-	-	10	10
Collateral systemic-to-pulmonary arteries	3	-	-	3
Trisomy 21	6 (6%)	**6 (35%)**	-	12 (10%)
Trisomy 13	3	-	-	3
Trisomy 18	3	-	-	3

*Associated defect.
AV, atrioventricular; *SVC*, superior vena cava, *VSD*, ventricular septal defect.

Coronary anomalies were noted in four cases: the origin of both the right and left coronary arteries from the right aortic sinus in one, origin of the anterior descending coronary artery from the right coronary artery in one and large infundibular branch running across the pulmonary infundibulum in two (Fig. 2.16).

Table 2.2 Associated extra cardiac anomalies in ToF in the Anatomical Collection of the University of Padua (20 cases)

Anomalies	N° cases	Anomalies	N° cases
Nervous system	7		
		Encephalocele	3
		Hydrocephalus	3
		Spina bifida	1
Gastrointestinal tract	17		
		Cleft lip and cleft palate	4
		Diaphragmatic hernia	1
		Esophageal atresia	1
		Duodenal stenosis	1
		Malrotation of the intestine	5
		Meckel's diverticulum	1
		Mesenterium commune	1
		Ano-rectal atresia	2
		Imperforate anus	1
Urinary system	6		
		Renal agenesis	3
		Horseshoe kidney	1
		Polycystic kidney	1
		Ureter duplication	1
Genital organs	5		
		Ambiguity of external genitalia	1
		Hypospadia	2
		Cryptorchidism	1
		Absent testis	1
Others	10		
		Aplasia cutis verticis	1
		Choanal atresia	1
		Microphthalmos or bulbar agenesis	2
		Coloboma	1
		Polydactyly-syndactyly	5

Extra cardiac anomalies (Table 2.2) were frequently present in patients who died young and particularly in association with chromosomal anomalies. From the review of the autopsy registry we found 20 cases with associated extra cardiac anomalies: 8 were fetal hearts, 11 infants (with ages ranging from 2 days to 10 months, median 1 month) and one was a 30-year-old male with left kidney agenesis. Trisomy 13 was found in two cases, trisomy 18 in two and trisomy 21 in one.

References

1. Fallot A (1888) Contribution a l'anatomie patologique de la maladie bleue (cyanose cardiaque). Marseille Med 25:77-93
2. Allwork SP (1988) Tetralogy of Fallot: the centenary of the name. A new translation of the first of Fallot's papers. Eur J Cardio Thorac Surg 2:368-392
3. Marquis RM (1956) Longevity and the early history of the tetralogy of Fallot. Br Med J 1:819-822
4. Stenonis N (1671-1672) Embryo monstro affinis Parisii dissectus. Acta Medica et Philosophica Hafniensia 1:200-203
5. Farre JR (1914) Pathological researches. Essay 1. On the malformation of the heart. Longman, Hurst, Rees, Orm and Brown, London, p 21
6. Peacock TB (1866) Malformation of the heart, 2 edn. Churchill, London 35:58-60
7. Von Rokitansky KF (1875) Die Defekte der Scheidewand des Herzens. Pathologisch-Anatomisch Wilhelm Braunmüller, Vienna, pp 27-29
8. Abbott ME, Dawson WT (1924) The clinical classification of congenital heart disease, with remarks upon its pathological anatomy, diagnosis and treatment. Int Clin 4:156-188
9. Abbott ME (1936) Atlas of congenital cardiac disease. Am Heart Association, New York, pp 46-47
10. Lev M, Eckner FAO (1964) The pathologic anatomy of tetralogy of Fallot and its variants. Dis Chest 45:251-261
11. Lev M, Rimoldi HJA, Rowlatt UF (1964) The quantitative anatomy of cyanotic tetralogy of Fallot. Circulation 30:531-538
12. Becker A, Connor M, Anderson RH (1975) Tetralogy of Fallot: a morphometric and geometric study. Am J Cardiol 35:402-412
13. Anderson RH, Allwork SP, Ho SY et al (1981) Surgical anatomy of tetralogy of Fallot. J Thorac Cardiovasc Surg 81:887-896
14. Anderson RH, Tynan M (1988) Tetralogy of Fallot – a centennial review. Int J Cardiol 21:219-232
15. Ho SY, Anderson RH (1990) The modern assessment of tetralogy of Fallot: morphological aspects. Chir Torac 43:101-110
16. Eisenmenger V (1897) Die angeborenen Defekte der Kammerscheidewand des Herzen. Z Klin Med 32:1-28
17. Oppenheimer-Dekker A, Gittenberger De Groot AC, Bartelings MM et al (1985) Abnormal architecture of the ventricles in hearts with an overriding aortic valve and a perimembranous ventricular septal defect ("Eisenmenger VSD"). Int J Cardiol 9:341-355
18. Anderson RH, Weinberg PM (2005) The clinical anatomy of tetralogy of Fallot. Cardiol Young 15:38-47
19. Anderson RH, Jacobs ML (2008) The anatomy of tetralogy of Fallot. Cardiol Young 18:12-21
20. Bailliard F, Anderson RH (2009) Tetralogy of Fallot. Orphanet J Rare Diseases 4:2-12
21. Van Praagh R, Van Praagh S, Nebesar RA et al (1970) Tetralogy of Fallot: underdevelopment of the pulmonary infundibulum and its sequelae. Am J Cardiol 26:25-33
22. Van Praagh R (1989) Etienne-Louis Arthur Fallot and his tetralogy: a new translation of Fallot's summary and a modern reassessment of this anomaly. Eur J Cardio-thorac Surg 3:381-386
23. Howell CE, Ho SY, Anderson RH, Elliott MJ (1990) Variation within the fibrous skeleton and ventricular outflow tracts in tetralogy of Fallot. Ann Thorac Surg 50:450-457
24. Anderson RH, Becker AE (1990) Etienne-Louis Arthur Fallot and his tetralogy: a new translation of Fallot's summary and a modern reassessment of this anomaly. Letter to Editor. Eur J Cardio-thorac Surg 4:229-230
25. Gatzoulis MA, Soukias N, Ho SY, Anderson RH (1990) Echocardiographic and morphological correlation in tetralogy of Fallot. Eur Heart J 20:221-231

26. Friedman BA, Hlavacek A, Chessa K et al (2010) Clinico-morphological correlations in the categorization of holes between the ventricles. Ann Ped Cardiol 3:12-24
27. Dickinson DF, Wilkinson JL, Smith A et al (1982) Variations in the morphology of the ventricular septal defect and disposition of the atrioventricular conduction tissues in tetralogy of Fallot. Thorac Cardiovasc Surg 30:243-249
28. Thiene G, Mazzucco A, Anderson RH et al (1984) Tetralogy of Fallot after surgery: autopsy review of 14 cases. Human Pathol 15:995-1018
29. Griffin ML, Sullivan ID, Anderson RH, McCartney FJ (1988) Doubly committed subarterial ventricular septal defect: new morphological criteria with ecocardiographic and angiographic correlation. Br Heart J 59:474-479
30. Thiene G, Bortolotti U, Gallucci V et al (1977) Pulmonary atresia with ventricular septal defect. Br Heart J 39: 1233-1240
31. Thiene G, Frescura C, Bini RM et al (1981) Histology of pulmonary arterial supply in pulmonary atresia with ventricular septal defect. Br Heart J 60:1066-1074
32. Anderson RH, Devine WA, Del Nido P (1991) The surgical anatomy of tetralogy of Fallot with pulmonary atresia rather than pulmonary stenosis. J Cardiac Surg 6:41-58
33. Ho YS, Catani A, Seo JW (1992) Arterial supply to the lungs in tetralogy of Fallot with pulmonary atresia or critical pulmonary stenosis. Cardiol Young 2:65-72
34. Thiene G, Frescura C, Di Donato R, Gallucci V (1979) Complete atrioventricular canal with conotruncal malformations: anatomical observations in 13 specimens. Europ J Cardiol 9:199-213
35. Bharati S, Kirklin JW, McAllister HA, Lev M (1980) The surgical anatomy of common atrioventricular orifice associated with tetralogy of Fallot, double outlet right ventricle and complete regular transposition. Circulation 61:1142-1149
36. Ricci M, Tchervenkov CI, Jacobs JP et al (2008) Surgical correction for patients with tetralogy of Fallot and common atrioventricular junction. Cardiol Young 18:29-38
37. Faggian G, Frescura C, Thiene G et al (1983) Accessory tricuspid valve tissue causing obstruction of the ventricular septal defect in tetralogy of Fallot. Br Heart J 49:318-324
38. Suzuki A, Ho YS, Anderson RH, Deanfield JE (1990) Further morphologic studies on tetralogy of Fallot with particular emphasis on the prevalence and structure of the membranous flap. J Thorac Cardiovasc Surg 99:528-535
39. Kurosawa H, Morita K, Yamagishi M et al (1998) Conotruncal repair for tetralogy of Fallot: midterm results. J Thorac Cardiovasc Surg 115:351-360
40. Emmanouilides GC, Thanopoulos B, Siassi B, Fishbein M (1976) "Agenesis" of ductus arteriosus associated with the syndrome of tetralogy of Fallot and absent pulmonary valve. Am J Cardiol 37:403-409
41. Rabinovitch M, Grady S, David I et al (1982) Compression of intrapulmonary bronchi by abnormally branching pulmonary arteries associated with absent pulmonary valve. Am J Cardiol 50:804-813
42. Milanesi O, Talenti E, Pellegrino PA, Thiene G (1984) Abnormal pulmonary artery branching in tetralogy of Fallot with absent pulmonary valve. Int J Cardiol 6:375-380
43. Velasquez G, Nath PH, Castaneda-Zuniga WR et al (1980) Aberrant left subclavian artery in tetralogy of Fallot. Am J Cardiol 45:811-818
44. Tan JL, Gatzoulis MA, Ho SY (2006) Aortic root disease in tetralogy of Fallot. Current opinion in Cardiology 2:569-572
45. Li J, Soukias ND, Carvalho JS, Ho SY (1988) Coronary arterial anatomy in tetralogy of Fallot: morphological and clinical correlation. Heart 80:74-183
46. Marino B, Digilio MC, Grazioli S et al (1996) Associated cardiac anomalies in isolated and syndromic patients with tetralogy of Fallot. Am J Cardiol 77:505-508
47. Momma K (2010) Cardiovascular anomalies associated with chromosome 22q11.2 deletion syndrome. Am J Cardiol 105:1617-1624
48. Kirklin JW, Blackstone EH, Kirklin JW et al (1981) Intracardiac surgery in infants under age 3 months: incremental risk factors for hospital mortality. Am J Cardiol 48:500-505
49. Lurz P, Bonhoeffer P, Taylor AM (2009) Percutaneous pulmonary valve implantation. An update. Expert Rev Cardiovasc Ther 7:823-833

50. Kirklin JW, McGoon DC, DuShane JW (1960) Surgical treatment of ventricular septal defect. J Thorac Cardiovasc Surg 40:763-770
51. Puga FJ, Leoni FE, Julsrud PR, Mair DD (1989) Complete repair of pulmonary atresia, ventricular septal defect and severe peripheral arborization abnormalities of the central pulmonary arteries: experience with preliminary unifocalazation procedures in 38 patients. J Thorac Cardiovasc Surg 98:1018-1029
52. Iyer KS, Mee RBB (1991) Staged repair of pulmonary atresia with ventricular septal defect and major systemic to pulmonary artery collaterals. Ann Thorac Cardiovasc Surg 51:62-72
53. Reddy MV, Liddicoat JR, Hanley FL (1995) Mid line one-stage complete unifocalization and repair of pulmonary atresia with ventricular septal defect and major aortopulmonary collaterals. J Thorac Cardiovasc Surg 109:832-845
54. Basso C, Frescura C, Corrado D et al (1995) Congenital heart disease and sudden death in the young. Human Pathol 26:1065-1072

Genetics

3

M. Cristina Digilio, Bruno Dallapiccola and Bruno Marino

3.1   Introduction

Genetics plays an important role in the etiology of congenital heart defects (CHDs), as demonstrated by clinical, epidemiological, embryological, and molecular studies. In fact, the finding of inherited CHDs, the association of CHDs with extracardiac defects and genetic syndromes and increasing knowledge about disease-associated genes are shedding light onto the role of genetic factors in determing CHDs.

Tetralogy of Fallot (ToF) represents about 60% of conotruncal heart defects. Extracardiac malformations in the setting of chromosomal or Mendelian syndromes are found in 25–35% of the patients with ToF [1–3]. Chromosomal anomalies are involved in 12% of the total cases, Mendelian syndromes or non-Mendelian associations in 7%, and non-classified multiple anomalies defects in 13% [1]. Disease genes have been identified in several syndromes, and in very few sporadic non-syndromic cases [4–10]. The correlation between anatomic cardiac patterns and some genetic anomalies suggests that specific morphogenetic mechanisms put in motion by genes can result in specific cardiac phenotypes [11].

3.2   Embryology

Recent embryological studies in chick and mouse embryo have delineated the contribution of the secondary heart field in the development of the outflow tract of the heart. The mammalian heart develops from a primary heart tube,

B. Marino (✉)
Pediatric Cardiology, Department of Pediatrics, Sapienza University, Rome, Italy
e-mail: bruno.marino@uniroma1.it

M. Chessa, A. Giamberti (eds.), *The Right Ventricle in Adults with Tetralogy of Fallot,*
© Springer-Verlag Italia 2012

which is formed by fusion of bilateral primary heart fields located in the lateral plate mesoderm. Earlier mapping studies of the heart fields in embryo cultures indicated that all of the myocardium of the developed heart originates from the primary heart field. Successive experiments in ovo suggested, on the contrary, that the atria, the majority of the right ventricle and conotruncus are added secondarily to the straight heart tube during looping [12]. Particularly, myocardium of the conotruncus is elongated from a midline secondary heart field of splanchnic mesoderm beneath the floor of the foregut [13–15]. The secondary heart field expresses genes fundamental in cardiac development, such as *Nkx2.5* and *GATA4*, prior to differentiation as myocardium, and cells are induced to become myocardium similar to the manner in which it occurs in the primary heart field. After neural crest ablation in the chick embryo, the myocardium is not added from the secondary heart field and the hearts have malaligned outflow tracts [16, 17]. Additionally, ablation of the secondary heart field in chick embryos leads to a subsets of CHDs that have overriding aorta and coronary artery anomalies, such as ToF with pulmonary atresia and double outlet right ventricle [18].

3.3 Syndromic Tetralogy of Fallot

3.3.1 Chromosomal Anomalies

Tetralogy of Fallot (ToF) can be associated with a great variety of chromosomal defects, and the most frequently diagnosed anomalies are trisomy 13 (Patau syndrome), trisomy 18 (Edwards syndrome) and trisomy 21 (Down syndrome) (Table 3.1) [19–21]. CHDs are present in about 80% of patients with trisomy 13 and 90% of children with trisomy 18. Anatomic types include classic ToF, VSD with polyvalvular dysplasia, atrial septal defect and double outlet right ventricle [19, 22].

Trisomy 21 (Down syndrome) is the most common identifiable cause of mental retardation with a prevalence of 1:700 live births. Atrioventricular canal defect (AVCD) is the commonest CHD in Down syndrome, while ToF is the only conotruncal anomaly described, occurring in 8% of the cases [21, 23]. As a distinctive anatomical characteristic, the ventricular septal defect (VSD) in patients with ToF and Down syndrome is particularly large, the subpulmonary stenosis is not usually severe, and the pulmonary arteries are usually good sized. Additionally, the only cardiac anomaly associated with ToF in trisomy 21 is the complete AVCD (Rastelli type C), sometimes with a hypoplastic right ventricle [23, 24]. Interestingly, cardiac defects sometimes associated with ToF in non-syndromic patients or those associated with different syndromes, like pulmonary atresia, absent pulmonary valve, discontinuity of pulmonary arteries, absent infundibular septum, are very rare in Down syndrome [21, 23].

Table 3.1 Clinical and cardiac characteristics of syndromes associated with ToF

Syndrome	Genetic defect	Extracardiac features	Subtype of ToF	Additional CHDs to ToF
Patau syndrome	Trisomy 13	Orofacial clefts Microphthalmia Aplasia cutis Polydactyly Growth deficiency Mental retardation	–	
Edwards syndrome	Trisomy 18	Facial anomalies Hand anomalies Cerebral anomalies Renal malformations Growth deficiency Mental retardation	–	Polyvalvular dysplasia
Down syndrome	Trisomy 21	Facial anomalies Duodenal stenosis Hirschsprung disease Hypotonia Mental retardation	Large VSD Good sized pulmonary arteries	Atrioventricular canal defect Hypoplastic right ventricle
Deletion 8p23	Deletion 8p23	Facial anomalies Microcephaly Hypospadia Mental retardation	–	Atrioventricular canal defect
DiGeorge/ Velo-cardio-facial syndrome	Deletion 22q11.2	Facial anomalies Palatal anomalies Neonatal hypocalcemia Immune deficit Speech defects Learning disabilities	Infundibular septum hypoplasia Pulmonary atresia	Aortic arch anomalies Aberrant left subclavian artery Absent pulmonary valve Hypoplasia of pulmonary arteries Major aorto-pulmonary collateral arteries

(cont.)

Table 3.1 (*continued*)

Alagille syndrome	JAG1 gene mutations Notch2 gene mutations	Chronic cholestasis Paucity of interlobular bile ducts Skeletal anomalies Ocular embryotoxon Facial anomalies	–	Multiple peripheral pulmonary artery stenosis
CHARGE syndrome	CHD7 gene mutations	Ocular coloboma Choanal atresia Ear anomalies Deafness Urogenital anomalies Growth retardation	–	Aortic arch anomalies Atrioventricular canal defect
VACTERL association	Unknown	Vertebral defects Anal atresia Esophageal atresia Renal anomalies Limb malformations	–	–
Oculo-Auriculo-Vertebral Spectrum (Goldenhar syndrome)	Unknown	Microtia Hemifacial microsomia Mandibular hypoplasia Epibulbar dermoid Cervical malformations	–	APVR

CHD, congenital heart defect; *VSD*, ventricular septal defect; *APVR*, anomalous pulmonary venous return.

Chromosomal imbalances involving chromosome 8 (8p23 deletion and recombinant 8 syndrome) are also chromosomal anomalies associated with ToF [25, 26]. Cardiac malformations are present in two third of these patients. The *GATA4* gene, which maps to the 8p23.1 region, is a candidate for CHD in del 8p23, being expressed in the developing heart [26, 27].

3.3.2 Microchromosomal Anomalies

Following advances in molecular/cytogenetic techniques, new chromosomal syndromes due to submicroscopic anomalies have been identified. Among them, 22q11.2 deletion syndrome, causing the phenotypical spectrum ranging from DiGeorge to Velo-Cardio-Facial syndrome, is the most frequent, with an estimated prevalence of approximately 1:4,000 live births. CHD is present in 75% of patients with 22q11.2 deletion syndrome [28, 29], classic ToF accounting for about 25% of them, and ToF with pulmonary atresia (PA) for an additional 25% [30]. On the contrary, 22q11.2 deletion syndrome is diagnosed in about 10% of patients with classic ToF [2, 31], and in about 35% of patients with pulmonary atresia with ventricular septal defect (PA-VSD) [3].

Patients with ToF and 22q11.2 deletion syndrome often have additional CHDs as a distinctive recognizable pattern. Additional cardiac defects are diagnosed in the half of the patients with classic ToF and 22q11.2 deletion syndrome [2, 30, 32]. The associated defects include: (1) right or cervical aortic arch with or without aberrant left subclavian artery; (2) hypoplasia or absence of the infundibular septum; (3) absence of the pulmonary valve; and (4) discontinuity or diffuse hypoplasia of the pulmonary arteries.

In regard to ToF with PA, the presence of major aorto-pulmonary collateral arteries, sometimes with discontinuity of the pulmonary arteries, is frequent in patients with 22q11.2 deletion syndrome [3, 33, 34]. These cases can be considered the true ToF with PA, with a prevalence of 22q11.2 deletion similar to that of patients with truncus arteriosus (35-40%) [3]. On the contrary, when PA-VSD is associated with ductus dependent pulmonary circulation and confluent pulmonary arteries, the frequency of 22q11.1 deletion is low, similar to that observed in patients with ToF (10%).

Deletion 22q11.2 syndrome is caused by a 3-megabase 22q11.2 deletion, containing just over 30 genes. The *TBX1* gene is mapping in the 22q11.2 critical region, and experimental animal studies have demonstrated that this gene is likely to be responsible for many heart and vascular anomalies in 22q11.2 deletion syndrome [35]. Interestingly, *TBX1* mutations have been rarely detected also in humans manifesting the DiGeorge/velo-cardio-facial syndrome facial and cardiac phenotype with or without mental retardation [36]. 22q11.2 deletion is exeptionally rare in patients with non-syndromic ToF [37], so that, in our opinion, screening for this deletion should be reserved for patients presenting with specific associated cardiovascular and/or extracardiac defects [38].

The new molecular technique of comparative genomic hybridization (CGH) is able to identify microchromosomal anomalies in 21% of patients with ToF [8]. Imbalances involve a great variety of chromosomal loci.

3.3.3 Monogenic Syndromes and Associations

Alagille syndrome is a genetically heterogeneous hepato-cardiac syndrome associated with CHD in up to 90% of patients, the most frequent being peripheral pulmonary stenosis. ToF is the most common complex cardiac malformation in these patients. A specific cardiovascular pattern has been described in this syndrome, consisting in the association of ToF with multiple and severe peripheral pulmonary artery stenosis [39]. Mutations in the *JAG1* gene, a ligand in the Notch signaling pathway, are responsible for Alagille syndrome in more than 90% of the cases. The study of the expression pattern of *JAG1* in the murine and human embryonic heart and vascular system demonstrated a correlation with the anatomic types of CHDs, since the gene is expressed prevalently at the arterial level [40]. Mutations in a second gene, *NOTCH2*, have been also identified in families segregating Alagille syndrome.

Additional genetic disorders known to be associated with ToF include CHARGE syndrome (for coloboma of the eye, heart defect, atresia choanae, retarded growth and development, genital hypoplasia and ear anomalies). CHD occurs in about 84% of patients with CHARGE syndrome, and ToF, sometimes associated with atrioventricular canal defect, is frequently detected [41]. Mutations in the *CHD7* gene cause the syndrome in the majority of these patients.

ToF is also often diagnosed in patients with association of malformations delineating a clinical entity without a specific detectable known genetic defect, known as VACTERL Association (for vertebral defects, anal atresia, cardiac defect, tracheo-esophageal fistula/esophageal atresia, renal anomalies, and limb malformations) [42], and the Oculo-Auriculo-Vertebral Spectrum (Goldenhar syndrome), characterized by microtia, hemifacial microsomia with mandibular hypoplasia, ocular epibulbar dermoid, and cervical vertebral malformations [43].

3.4 Non-syndromic Patients

Non-syndromic ToF is genetically heterogeneous, the number of identified genes is low, and molecular analysis of large series of patients has shown that each single gene defect is detectable in a few cases (Table 3.2). The identified disease genes point to a key role for transcription factors in the process of cardiac maldevelopment. Among candidate genes, *NKX2.5* is expressed in early cardiac mesoderm, and mutation in mice leads to failure of cardiac development at the linear heart tube stage. *NKX2.5* gene mutations have been detected in 1–4% of non-syndromic ToF [4, 6, 8]. *NKX2.5* participates at the molec-

Table 3.2 Gene mutations in non-syndromic ToF

Gene	Mutated patients/ analyzed patients	%	Reference
NKX2.5	6/150	4%	Goldmuntz et al. [4]
	9/201	4.5%	McElhinney et al. [6]
	2/194	1%	Rauch et al. [8]
FOG2	2/47	4%	Pizzuti et al. [7]
CITED2	3/46	6%	Sperling et al. [44]
NODAL pathway	15/121	12%	Roessler et al. [5]
JAG1	3/94	3%	Bauer et al. [9]
	3/112	2.7%	Guida et al. [10]
TBX1 variants	3/93	3%	Griffin et al. [45]
	2/191	1%	Rauch et al. [8]
FOXA2	4/93	4%	Topf et al. [46]
GJA5	2/178	1%	Guida et al. [47]
FOXC1	1/93	1%	Topf et al. [46]
HAND2	1/93	1%	Topf et al. [46]

ular level in protein interactions with at least two other important cardiac transcription factors, *GATA4* and *TBX5*. *FOG2* is the likely mediator of *GATA4* cardiac developmental defects, and is mutated in 4% of non-syndromic ToF patients [7]. Mice lacking the transcription factor *CITED2* have CHDs causing in utero death, and *CITED2* mutations have been detected in 6% of ToF in humans [44]. Mutations in one of the genes causing Alagille syndrome, *JAG1*, have also been detected in patients with non-syndromic ToF, in about 3% of the cases [9, 10]. Mutations in components of the human NODAL-signaling pathway have also been documented in patients with ToF [5]. Studies have demonstrated that rare TBX1 variants are present in a small percentage of non-syndromic TOF [8, 45].

Very recent contributions show new variants in *FOXC1, HAND2, FOXA2* [46] and in *GJA5* gene [47] in humans with ToF. Nevertheless, it should be considered that in some instances genetic variations found in the probands were also present in their unaffected parents, possibly being considered as susceptibility factors and not an unique cause of ToF.

Several copy number variations (CNVs) have also been recently identified in non-syndromic sporadic ToF patients [8, 48-50], corresponding to chromosomal loci with known disease-associated genes (*NOTCH1, JAG1, GJA5*), but also to new critical regions possibly corresponding to new genes for CHD. The results reported by Greenway et al. [48] predict that at least 10% of sporadic non-syndromic patients with ToF can result from de novo CNVs, and suggest that mutations in gene located within these loci might be etiologic in other cases of ToF.

3.5   Recurrence Risks and Genetic Counseling

In practical genetic counseling, empiric risk figures are used in order to calculate the recurrence risks for subsequent pregnancies of couples with a child with ToF. In fact, healthy non-consanguineous parents of a child affected by ToF have a recurrence risk for CHD corresponding to 3% [51]. The risk is higher when additional relatives are affected. Particularly, if two siblingss are affected, the recurrence risk of the couple corresponds to 10%. In the largest study of recurrence risks using a population-based registry of adult survivors with significant CHDs, the recurrence risk among offspring of affected patients corresponded to 4.1% [52].

3.6   Genotype-prognosis Correlations

Patients with ToF and an associated genetic syndrome represent a challenge to the cardiac surgeon, who must consider issues from the possible need for extracardiac surgery on associated malformations, to the presence of immunodeficiency or altered compliance of the pulmonary vasculature [53]. The study of the outcome of surgical correction of classic ToF in syndromic and non-syndromic patients, including several different syndromic conditions, shows that 22q11.2 deletion does not represent a surgical risk factor. However, genetic syndromes different from 22q11.2 deletion and Down syndromes, particularly VACTERL Association, have an important negative impact on surgical outcome of CHD [54, 55]. Risk factors for mortality in this group of patients included pulmonary artery hypoplasia and surgical repair of extracardiac anomalies, possibly leading to secondary changes in pulmonary compliance and pulmonary mechanics, and to an increased incidence of gram negative infections. However, in patients with ToF and pulmonary atresia (PA with VSD) the presence of 22q11.2 deletion is associated with an high surgical mortality, probably due to the complexity of the pulmonary artery anatomy [56, 57].

3.7   Conclusion

The general phenotype of ToF may be associated with multiple genetic causes, and may involve different pathogenetic mechanisms. In relation to specific genetic causes and pathogenetic mechanisms, the phenotype may present specific characteristics. For example, ToF associated with trisomy 21 seems to have "myocardial origin", and is characterized by large VSD and good sized pulmonary arteries. In patients with ToF and deletion of 22q11.2, the pathogenetic mechanism involves the secondary heart field [18], and the phenotype includes anomalies of the aortic arch, pulmonary arteries, infundibular septum and pulmonary valve. ToF in patients with Alagille syndrome and mutations in the *JAG1* gene are probably in relation to a primary involvement of the pulmonary arteries, since this gene is expressed only in the pulmonary arteries, and these frequently show multiple peripheral stenosis [39].

Different genetic anomalies and different pathogenetic mechanisms may cause similar phenotypic defects, which we call, in general, ToF. Detailed diagnosis is essential not only for genetic assessment, but also to guide surgical treatment and perioperative prognosis.

References

1. Ferencz C, Loffredo CA, Correa-Villasenor A, Wilson PD (1997) Genetic and environmental risk factors of major cardiovascular malformations. The Baltimore-Washington Infant Study 1981-1989. Futura Publishing Company Inc, Armonk, New York
2. Marino B, Digilio MC, Grazioli S et al (1996) Associated cardiac anomalies in isolated and syndromic patients with tetralogy of Fallot. Am J Cardiol 77:505-508
3. Digilio MC, Marino B, Grazioli S et al (1996) Comparison of occurrence of genetic syndromes in ventricular septal defect with pulmonic stenosis (classic tetralogy of Fallot) versus ventricular septal defect with pulmonic atresia. Am J Cardiol 77:1375-1376
4. Goldmuntz E, Geiger E, Benson W (2001) NKX2.5 mutations in patients with tetralogy of Fallot. Circulation 104:2565-2568
5. Roessler E, Ouspenskaia MV, Karkera JD et al (2008) Reduced NODAL signaling strength via mutation of several pathway members including FOXH1 is linked to human heart defects and holoprosencephaly. Am J Hum Genet 83:18-29
6. McElhinney DB, Geiger E, Blinder J et al (2003) Nkx2.3 mutations in patients with congenital heart disease. J Am Coll Cardiol 42:1650-1655
7. Pizzuti A, Sarkozy A, Newton AL et al (2003) Mutations in ZFPM2/FOG2 gene in sporadic cases of tetralogy of Fallot. Hum Genet 22:372-377
8. Rauch R, Hofbeck M, Zweier C et al (2010) Comprehensive genotype-phenotype analysis in 230 patients with tetralogy of Fallot. J Med Genet 47:321-331
9. Bauer RC, Laney AO, Smith R et al (2010) Jagged1 (JAG1) mutations in patients with tetralogy of Fallot or pulmonic stenosis. Hum Mutation 31:594-601
10. Guida V, Chiappe F, Ferese R et al (2011) Novel and recurrent JAG1 mutations in patients with tetralogy of Fallot. Clin Genet 80:591-594
11. Marino B, Digilio MC (2000) Congenital heart disease and genetic syndromes: Correlation between cardiac phenotype and genotype. Cardiovasc Pathol 9:303-315
12. de la Cruz MV, Sanchez Gomez C, Arteaga MM, Arguello C (1977) Experimental study of the development of the truncus and the conus in the chick embryo. J Anat 123:661-686
13. Waldo KL, Kumiski DH, Wallis KT et al (2001) Conotruncal myocardium arises from a secondary heart field. Development 128:3179-3188
14. Mjaatvedt CH, Nakaoka T, Moreno-Rodriguez R et al (2001) The outflow tract of the heart is recruited from a novel heart-forming field. Developmental Biol 238:97-109
15. Zaffran S, Kelly RG, Meilhac SM et al (2004) Right ventricular myocardium derives from the anterior heart field. Circ Res 95:261-268
16. Yelbuz TM, Waldo KL, Kumuski DH et al (2002) Shortened outflow tract leads to altered cardiac looping after neural crest ablation. Circulation 106:504-510
17. Waldo KL, Hutson MR, Stadt HA et al (2005) Cardial neural crest is necessary for normal addition of the myocardium to the arterial pole from the secondary heart field. Dev Biol 281:66-77
18. Ward C, Stadt H, Hutson M, Kirby ML (2005) Ablation of the secondary heart field leads to tetralogy of Fallot and pulmonary atresia. Developmental Biol 284:72-83

19. Musewe NN, Alexander DJ, Teshima I et al (1990) Echocardiographic evaluation of the spectrum of cardiac anomalies associated with trisomy 18 and 13. J Am Coll Cardiol 15:673-677

20. Karr SS, Brenner JI, Loffredo C et al (1992) Tetralogy of Fallot. The spectrum of severity in a regional study, 1981-1985. Am J Dis Child 146:121-124

21. Marino B (1996) Patterns of congenital heart disease and associated cardiac anomalies in children with Down syndrome. In: Marino B, Pueschel SM (eds) Heart disease in persons with Down syndrome. Brookes, Baltimore, pp 33-40

22. Van Praagh S, Truman T, Firpo A et al (1989) Cardiac malformations in trisomy 18: A study of 41 postmortem cases. J Am Coll Cardiol 13:1586-1597

23. Marino B (1993) Congenital heart disease in patients with Down's syndrome: anatomic and genetic aspects. Biomed & Pharmacother 47:197-200

24. Vergara P, Digilio MC, De Zorzi A et al (2006) Genetic heterogeneity and phenotypic anomalies in children with atrioventricular canal defect and tetralogy of Fallot. Clin Dysmorphol 15:65-70

25. Digilio MC, Marino B, Guccione P et al (1998) Deletion 8p sindrome. Am J Med Genet 75:534-536

26. Giglio S, Graw SL, Gimelli G et al (2000) Deletion of a 5-cM region at chromosome 8p23 is associated with a spectrum of congenital heart defects. Circulation 102:432-437

27. Devriendt K, Matthijs G, Van Dael R et al (1999) Delineation of the critical deletion region for congenital heart defects, on chromosome 8p23.1. Am J Hum Genet 64:1119-1126

28. Ryan AK, Goodship JA, Wilson DI et al (1997) Spectrum of clinical features associated with interstitial chromosome 22q11 deletions: a European collaborative study. J Med Genet 34:798-804

29. McDonald-McGinn DM, Kirschner R, Goldmuntz E et al (1999) The Philadelphia story. The 22q11.2 deletion: report on 250 patients. Genet Couns 10:11-24

30. Marino B, Digilio MC, Toscano A et al (2001) Anatomic patterns of conotruncal defects associated with deletion 22q11. Genet Med 3:45-48

31. Goldmuntz E, Clark BJ, Mitchell LE et al (1998) Frequency of 22q11 deletions in patients with conotruncal defects. J Am Coll Cardiol 32:492-498

32. Momma K, Kondo C, Ando M et al (1995) Tetralogy of Fallot associated with chromosome 22q11 deletion. Am J Cardiol 76:618-621

33. Momma K, Kondo C, Matsuoka R (1996) Tetralogy of Fallot with pulmonary atresia associated with chromosome 22q11 deletion. J Am Coll Cardiol 27:198-202

34. Anaclerio S, Marino B, Carotti A et al (2001) Pulmonary atresia with ventricular septal defect: prevalence of deletion 22q11 in the different anatomic patterns. Ital Heart J 2:384-387

35. Lindsay EA, Vitelli F, Su H et al (2001) Tbx1 haploinsufficiency in the DiGeorge syndrome region causes aortic arch defects in mice. Nature 410:97-101

36. Yagi H, Furutani Y, Hamada H et al (2003) Role of TBX1 in human del22q11.2 syndrome. Lancet 362:1366-1373

37. Amati F, Mari A, Digilio MC et al (1995) 22q11 deletions in isolated and syndromic patients with tetralogy of Fallot. Hum Genet 95:479-482

38. Digilio MC, Marino B, Giannotti A et al (1999) Guidelines for 22q11 deletion screening of patients with conotruncal defects. J Am Coll Cardiol 33:1746-1747

39. McElhinney DB, Krantz ID, Bason L et al (2002) Analysis of cardiovascular phenotype and genotype-phenotype correlation in individuals with a JAG1 mutation and/or Alagille syndrome. Circulation 106:2567-2574

40. Loomes KM, Underkoffler LA, Morabito et al (1999) The expression of JAGGED1 in the developing mammalian heart correlates with cardiovascular disease in Alagille syndrome. Hum Molec Genet 8:2443-2449

41. Trip J, van Stuijvenberg M, Dikkers FG, Pijnenburg MW (2002) Unilateral CHARGE association. Eur J Pediatr 161:78-80

42. Botto L, Khoury MJ, Mastroiacovo P et al (1997) The spectrum of congenital anomalies of the VATER association: An international study. Am J Med Genet 71:8-15

43. Digilio MC, Calzolari F, Capolino R et al (2008) Congenital heart defects in patients with Oculo-Auriculo-Vertebral spectrum (Goldenhar syndrome). Am J Med Genet 146A:1815-1819

44. Sperling S, Grimm CH, Dunkel I et al (2005) Identification and functional analysis of CITED2 mutations in patients with congenital heart defects. Hum Mutation 26:575-582

45. Griffin HR, Topf A, Glen E et al (2010) Systematic survey of variants in TBX1 in non-syndromic tetralogy of Fallot identifies a novel 57 base pair deletion that reduces transcriptional activity but finds no evidence for association with common variants. Heart 96:1651-1655

46. Topf A, Griffin HR, Hall DH et al (2011) Gene screening of the secondary heart field network in tetralogy of Fallot patients. Heart 97(Suppl 1):A76 (Abstract)

47. Guida V, Ferese R, Rocchetti M et al (2012) A variant in the carboxyl-terminus of connexin 40 alters GAP junctions and increases risk for tetralogy of Fallot (submitted)

48. Greenway SC, Pereira AC, Lin JC et al (2009) De novo copy number variants identify new genes and loci in isolated sporadic tetralogy of Fallot. Nat Genet 41:931-935

49 Wang J, Xie XD, Zhou S et al (2011) The study of copy number variations in the regions of NOTCH1 among Chinese and TOF patients. Int J Cardiol 14:444-484

50. Soemedi R, Topf A, Wilson IJ et al (2011) Phenotype-specific effect of chromosome 1q21.1 rearrangements and GJA5 duplications in 2436 congenital heart disease patients and 6760 controls. Hum Molec Genet (E-pub ahead of printing)

51. Digilio MC, Marino B, Giannotti A et al (1997) Recurrence risk figures for isolated tetralogy of Fallot after screening for 22q11 microdeletion. J Med Genet 34:188-190

52. Burn J, Brennan P, Little H et al (1998) Recurrence risks in offspring of adults with major heart defect: results from first cohort of British collaborative study. Lancet 351:311-316

53. Formigari R, Michielon G, Digilio MC et al (2009) Genetic syndromes and congenital heart defects: how is surgical management affected? Eur J Cardio-Thorac Surg 35:606-614

54. Michielon G, Marino B, Formigari R et al (2006) Genetic syndromes and outcome after surgical correction of tetralogy of Fallot. Ann Thorac Surg 81:968-975

55. Michielon G, Marino B, Oricchio G et al (2009) Impact of Del22q11, trisomy 21, and other genetic syndromes on surgical outcome of conotruncal heart defects. J Thorac Cardiovasc Surg 138:565-570

56. Carotti A, Marino B, Di Donato RM (2003) Influence of chromosome 22q11.2 microdeletion on surgical outcome after treatment of tetralogy of Fallot with pulmonary atresia. J Thorac Cardiovasc Surg 126:1666-1667

57. Carotti A, Albanese SB, Filippelli S (2010) Determinants of outcome after surgical treatment of pulmonary atresia with ventricular septal defect and major aortopulmonary collateral arteries. J Thorac Cardiovasc Surg 140:1092-1103

Stem Cells and the Right Ventricle

4

Luigi Anastasia and Marco Piccoli

4.1 Introduction

Stem cell research has been one of the most investigated fields by the scientific community in the past decade. This unprecedented attention has been mainly caused by the number of possible applications of stem cells in regenerative medicine, which has created expectations of curing widespread diseases like Parkinson's, Alzheimer's, and heart failure. In particular, regenerating the heart, which is one of the least regenerative organs of the body, has been an incredible challenge. However, recent discoveries have proven that also the heart is a self-renewing organ characterized by resident cardiac stem cells (CSCs) stored in niches [1]. This revolutionary view of the heart raises the possibility that defects in myocardial homeostasis and ventricular dysfunction occur because of a progressive increase in the number of CSCs permanently withdrawn from the cell cycle [2]. The rate of accumulation of old CSCs might be greater than the rate of their death and replacement, leading to the formation of senescent niches and organ aging. Moreover, the recognition that the heart possesses a stem cell compartment, which has been shown to regenerate myocytes and coronary vessels both in vitro and in vivo in animal models, supports the notion that it is indeed possible to reconstitute dead myocardium after infarction, to repopulate the hypertrophic decompensated heart with new myocytes and vascular structures, and perhaps to reverse ventricular dilation and wall thinning, restoring the physiological and anatomical characteristics of the normal heart [3–5].

L. Anastasia (✉)
Department of Medical Chemistry, Biochemistry and Biotechnology, University of Milan, Italy;
IRCCS Policlinico San Donato, San Donato Milanese (Mi), Italy

M. Chessa, A. Giamberti (eds.), *The Right Ventricle in Adults with Tetralogy of Fallot,*
© Springer-Verlag Italia 2012

4.2   Stem Cell Types and Therapeutic Applications

While advances in the prevention and early treatment of atherosclerotic heart disease have reduced cardiovascular morbidity, once damage to the heart has occurred, present therapies only rarely result in long-term improvement of cardiac function [6]. Therefore, despite the use of new therapies, the prognosis of patients with heart failure is generally unfavorable. Great expectations reside in regenerative medicine, especially due to the promise of new stem cell therapies. However, myocardial infarction results in large-scale loss of cardiac muscle (often a billion or more myocytes), therefore a cell-based therapy, to be feasible, needs to start from large numbers of progenitor cells. Therefore, the use of embryonic stem cells (ES cells), which can be easily expanded to large numbers, initially seemed to be the right choice. Unfortunately, ES cells not only raise ethical concerns, but suffer from intrinsic difficulties, as their fate is still very tricky to direct, and they are also prone to form teratomas [7]. However, in recent years, a new promising approach has surfaced, consisting of the possibility of reprogramming somatic cells (adult cells) into stem cell-like progenitors [8–10]. Different experimental approaches have been used, including somatic cell nuclear transfer, cloning (with a very low success rate), cell fusion of somatic cells with ES cells, ectopic gene expression and/or treatment with exogenous factors. More recently, it has been shown that the combined expression of some transcription factors, known to be involved in stem cell self-renewal, can reprogram mouse fibroblasts to pluripotent cells [11]. These cells, called induced Pluripotent Stem Cells (iPSCs), are almost indistinguishable from ES cells [10]. Unfortunately, iPSCs may suffer the same problems of ES cells, as some of them tend to degenerate into tumors [12]. It is clear that a much deeper understanding of the molecular and developmental processes that are involved in stem cell fate regulation is mandatory in order to govern the reprogramming of somatic cells and that novel experimental approaches need to be researched. Thus many leading groups involved in stem cell research have speculated that a chemical approach may circumvent these problems, but this field is still at its early stages. However, this approach may ultimately provide chemical drugs that would help generate stem cell-like progenitors from easily accessible and abundant adult cells, which are intrinsically safer than genetically modified cells [13]. In fact, chemical induction/reprogramming has several intrinsic advantages over genetic manipulation: (1) avoiding the possible tumoral degeneration following genome perturbation; (2) timing, as drugs can usually reach their target(s) very quickly and selectively; (3) control, as the concentration of the drug can be easily varied to reach the desired effect in the most efficient way; (4) simplicity, as chemical treatments will allow a very simple tool, as compared to the use of retro- or lenti-viral systems; and (5) low cost, as new drugs, once identified, can be easily synthesized in large scale by consolidated methods [14]. For example a synthetic purine named reversine, which was identified by a high-throughput screening of a combinatorial library, was shown to revert mouse proliferating myoblasts to a more undifferentiated state, similar to stem cells [8]. Reversine is also able to induce the de-differentiation of human dermal fibroblasts, which can then be induced to differentiate into skeletal and smooth muscle cells and bone [9]. Although reversine treatment led to up-regulation of priming genes of neuroectodermal lineages, such as *Ngn2*, *Nts*, *Irx3*, *Pax7*, *Hes1*, and *Hes6*, through active histone modifications in the promoter regions of these genes, the reprogramming mechanism induced by the molecule is yet to be clarified. However, initial results seem to indicate that the molecule interacts with key proteins involved in cytoskeletal and cell shape remodeling, RNA export, degradation, folding, stress control and ATP production [15].

Finding a safe and efficient way of generating stem cells is only half the battle. In fact, once progenitors cells are made, it is crucial to have very selective and high yielding methods to pilot their differentiation toward the desired cell phenotype. Besides the use of ES cells or iPSCs, which is still very problematic, adult stem cells can normally be differentiated into a limited number of cell types, usually inherent to the tissue where they reside. However, while many successful differentiations have been reported in the literature, especially in the case of mesenchymal cells, we are still far from highly efficient differentiation methods, as would be required for an effective therapeutic tool. Moreover, in vitro and in vivo behavior of stem cells is often different, and most studies do not possess an animal study counterpart, so they are difficult to judge. Although each different type of adult stem cell should be considered alone, there are some general problems associated with their use: (1) they can be obtained in very small numbers from adult individuals; (2) they can only be grown for a limited number of passages in vitro before losing their differentiation potential; (3) the yields of differentiation are often too low to be practical for therapeutic use. As in the case of ES cells, differentiation of adult stem cells is obtained ex vivo with cocktails of growth factors and signaling molecules. Furthermore, some recently discovered adult stem cells, like neural stem cells (NSCs) or cardiac progenitor cells, possess a very limited turnover, thus new chemically defined growth conditions are needed. Along these lines, it has been reported that a synthetic sulfonylhydrazone (Shz-1), found in a combinatorial library screen for the activation of *Nkx2.5*, can trigger cardiac differentiation of human mobilized peripheral blood mononuclear cells (M-PBMCc), and these in vitro generated human cardiac cells can engraft into a rat heart in proximity to an experimental injury, improving cardiac function [16], and very recently were used to induce the cardiac differentiation of iPSCs [17]. However, if the adult heart possesses a pool of primitive multipotent cells, these cells may be the most reliable and therapeutically safest choice, before more complex and unknown cells are explored. The attraction of this approach is its intrinsic simplicity. In fact, cardiac regeneration would be accomplished by enhancing the normal turnover of myocardial cells. Along this line, several investigators have reported resident population of cardiac stem cells (CSCs), which were identified using a variety of approaches [18]. CSCs expressing the tyrosine kinase receptor c-kit are by far the most extensively studied [3]. In the adult, c-kit is expressed by telocytes, the thymic epithelium and mature circulating cells such as hematopoietic stem cells and mast cells. Immature endothelial cells and cardiomyocytes also express c-kit during development [19]. Cells expressing c-kit have been identified in the perivascular compartment of the adult heart, and their abundance increases in human heart failure [20]. They have been reported to give rise to cardiomyocytes, smooth muscle cells and endothelial cells. Moreover, the surface antigens c-kit, MDR1 or Sca-1 are present in cells undergoing lineage differentiation, complicating recognition of the actual primitive cells in the population [9]. CSCs are lineage negative primitive cells expressing only the surface antigens c-kit, MDR1 and Sca-1 protein alone or in combination [21]. CSCs are negative for transcription factors present in cardiac cells, GATA-4 and GATA-5; myocytes, Nkx2.5 and MEF2C; ECs, Ets1 and Erg1; SMCs, GATA-6; skeletal muscle cells, MyoD, myogenin and Myf5; and hematopoietic cells, GATA-2 and GATA-3. CSCs are also negative for cytoplasmic proteins specific for myocytes (nestin, desmin and cardiac myosin heavy chain, α-sarcomeric actin, connexin 43 and N-cadherin), ECs (CD34, CD31, von Willebrand factor and flk1), SMCs (TGFβ1 receptor, flk1 and α-smooth muscle actin), neural cells (MAP1b, neurofilament 200 and GFAP), and hematopoietic cells (CD45, CD45RO, CD8, CD20 and TER 119) [3]. Progenitor cells express stem cell antigens and transcription factors of cardiac cell lineages or, more specifically, of myocytes, ECs and SMCs. Progenitor cells do not express specific cytoplasmic proteins. Precursor cells exhibit stem cell antigens in combination with cytoplasmic proteins typical of myocytes, ECs or SMCs. On the basis of these data, a clinical trial is under way, testing the safety and feasibility of autologous c-kit[+] cells as an adjunctive treatment for patients undergoing coronary bypass surgery (ClinicalTrials.gov, identifier NCT00474461). CSCs are isolated, expanded in vitro and then re-injected (Fig. 4.1). So far, other experimental studies and clinical trials have employed rather heterogeneous bone marrow cell preparations in an attempt to regenerate dead myocardium after infarction. Actually, considerable interest in bone-marrow-derived cells for cardiac repair was prompted by reports of hematopoietic stem cells transdifferentiating into cardiomyocytes [22]. With a few exceptions [23, 24], the injection of bone marrow cells has resulted in a consistent improvement in function of the infarcted heart in both animals and humans [22, 25]. However, these reports have not answered the critical question of whether one bone marrow cell has a more powerful therapeutic efficacy than another. It is hard to envision that any cell of bone marrow origin can form new myocardium with functionally competent myocytes and coronary vessels. In the majority of cases, the administered cells were not characterized and, most likely, represented a combination of therapeutically effective and non-effective cells. Importantly, cells with distinct epitopes were not tested, and paracrine signaling as the major mechanism of action has also been speculated. Mesenchymal stem cells (MSCs) are also in clinical trials (NCT00587990). There are several reports with these cells, but one of the strongest cardiac-repair treatment effects seen was obtained

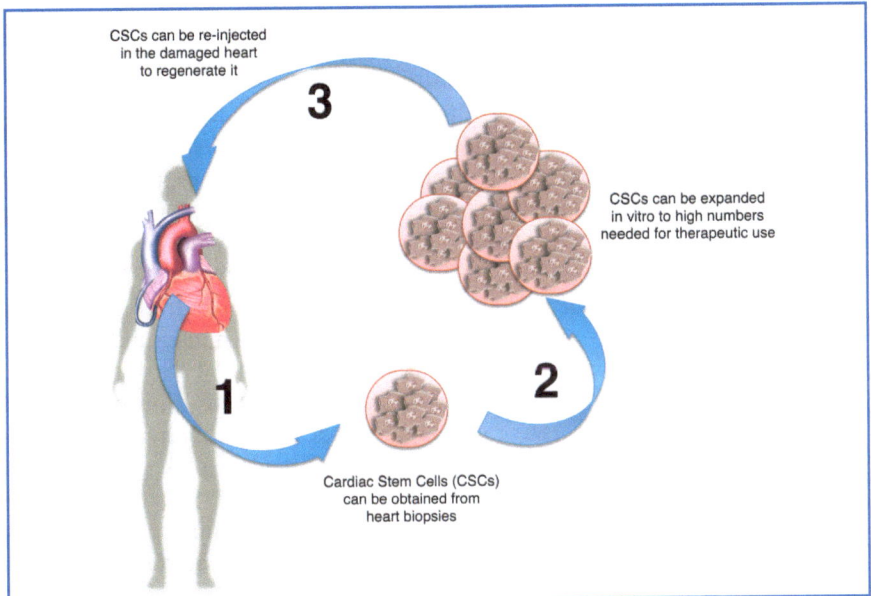

CSCs can be re-injected in the damaged heart to regenerate it

3

CSCs can be expanded in vitro to high numbers needed for therapeutic use

1

2

Cardiac Stem Cells (CSCs) can be obtained from heart biopsies

Fig. 4.1 Cell therapy approach to cardiac regeneration with endogenous CSCs

after the intracoronary administration of large numbers of autologous MSCs [26]. Allogeneic MSCs administered to patients intravenously within 10 days of infarction were well tolerated and were associated with decreased arrhythmias and an improvement in some indices of contractile function [27].

4.3 Applications in the Right Ventricle and Future Developments

For many years emphasis in cardiology and, consequently, in regenerative medicine was mainly on the left ventricle (LV), overshadowing the study of the right ventricle (RV). However, more recently, cardiac surgeons recognized the importance of the RV in heart failure, RV myocardial infarction, congenital heart disease and pulmonary hypertension. Along these lines, the stem cell community has started to look into RV pathologies to find new possible therapeutic opportunities with stem cells. For example, ToF is now considered a genetic disorder that is frequently found in association with trisomy 21, and the current view is that a genetic defect of cardiac stem cells may cause the malformations that occur in ToF [28]. Point mutations identified in patients with ToF support the hypothesis that this syndrome may be a result of altered proliferation, differentiation and migration of the precardiac cells of the secondary heart field during heart development. Clearly the understanding of the mechanisms underlying the migration and proliferation of CSCs in patients with ToF is key to developing new possible stem-cell-based surgical approaches for this disease that for instance may reduce the incidence of late sudden death in these patients. Recently, evaluation has been carried out of the feasibility and efficacy of autologous umbilical cord blood mononuclear cell (UCMNC) transplantation on right ventricular (RV) function in a novel sheep animal model of chronic RV volume overload, which is the most dominant factor contributing to late morbidity and mortality of ToF patients [29]. Results indicate that the chronically volume-overloaded RV profits from autologous UCMNC implantation by enhanced diastolic properties with a probable underlying mechanism of increased angiogenesis. Similar to ToF, arrhythmogenic right ventricular cardiomyopathy (ARVC) has very recently been recognized as a cardiac stem cell disease [30]. Mechanistic studies indicate that suppressed canonical Wnt signaling [31], imposed by nuclear plakoglobin, is the mechanism responsible for the pathogenesis of ARVC. This causes a subset of second heart field cardiac progenitor cells in the epicardium to differentiate into adipocytes due to enhanced expression of adipogenic factors. This mechanism explains the predominant involvement of the right ventricle in ARVC [28]. The very recent discovery that functionally competent CSCs can be isolated from endomyocardial biopsies creates a new opportunity for an easily accessible source of autologous stem cells to develop future therapies for patients with advanced cardiomyopathies [32]. It is undoubtedly clear that stem cell therapies will dominate the next decade or two, and only time will tell how many different cardiac diseases will be suitable for this therapeutic approach. It is not difficult to foresee that once stem cell therapies become available, they will be initially accompanied by drug treatments to support and improve stem cell survival, migration and differentiation, after cell implantation. Further ahead, new drugs may be developed to activate cardiac stem cells in situ, without the need for cell isolation, expansion in the laboratory and re-implantation. This is where a chemico-pharmacological approach to stem cell biology will become crucial.

References

1. Urbanek K, Cesselli D, Rota M et al (2006) Stem cell niches in the adult mouse heart. Proc Natl Acad Sci USA 103:9226-9231
2. Cesselli D, Beltrami AP, D'Aurizio F et al (2011) Effects of age and heart failure on human cardiac stem cell function. Am J Pathol 179:349-366
3. Bearzi C, Rota M, Hosoda T et al (2007) Human cardiac stem cells. Proc Natl Acad Sci USA 104:14068-4073
4. Bearzi C, Leri A, Lo Monaco F et al (2009) Identification of a coronary vascular progenitor cell in the human heart. Proc Natl Acad Sci USA 106:15885-90
5. Rota M, Padin-Iruegas ME, Misao Y et al (2008) Local activation or implantation of cardiac progenitor cells rescues scarred infarcted myocardium improving cardiac function. Circ Res 103:107-116

6. Jessup M, Brozena S (2003) Heart failure. N Engl J Med 348:2007-2018
7. Blum B, Benvenisty N (2008) The tumorigenicity of human embryonic stem cells. Adv Cancer Res 100:133-158
8. Chen S, Zhang Q, Wu X et al (2004) Dedifferentiation of lineage-committed cells by a small molecule. J Am Chem Soc 126:410-401
9. Anastasia L, Sampaolesi M, Papini N et al (2006) Reversine-treated fibroblasts acquire myogenic competence in vitro and in regenerating skeletal muscle. Cell Death Differ 13:2042-2051
10. Takahashi K, Yamanaka S (2006) Induction of pluripotent stem cells from mouse embryonic and adult fibroblast cultures by defined factors. Cell 126:663-676
11. Noisa P, Parnpai R (2011) Technical challenges in the derivation of human pluripotent cells. Stem Cells Int 2011:907-961
12. Ben-David U, Benvenisty N, Mayshar Y (2010) Genetic instability in human induced pluripotent stem cells: classification of causes and possible safeguards. Cell Cycle 9:4603-4604
13. Anastasia L, Pelissero G, Venerando B, Tettamanti G (2010) Cell reprogramming: expectations and challenges for chemistry in stem cell biology and regenerative medicine. Cell Death Differ 17:1230-1237
14. Anastasia L, Piccoli M, Garatti A et al (2011) Cell reprogramming: a new chemical approach to stem cell biology and tissue regeneration. Curr Pharm Biotechnol 12:146-150
15. Fania C, Anastasia L, Vasso M et al (2009) Proteomic signature of reversine-treated murine fibroblasts by 2-D difference gel electrophoresis and MS: Possible associations with cell signalling networks. Electrophoresis 30:2193-2206
16. Sadek H, Hannack B, Choe E et al (2008) Cardiogenic small molecules that enhance myocardial repair by stem cells. Proc Natl Acad Sci U S A 105:6063-6068
17. Quattrocelli M, Palazzolo G, Agnolin I et al (2011) Synthetic sulfonyl-hydrazone-1 positively regulates cardiomyogenic microRNA expression and cardiomyocyte differentiation of induced pluripotent stem cells. J Cell Biochem 112:2006-2014
18. Laflamme MA, Murry CE (2011) Heart regeneration. Nature 473:326-335
19. Tallini YN, Greene KS, Craven M et al (2009) c-kit expression identifies cardiovascular precursors in the neonatal heart. Proc Natl Acad Sci U S A 106:1808-1813
20. Kubo H, Jaleel N, Kumarapeli A et al (2008) Increased cardiac myocyte progenitors in failing human hearts. Circulation 118:649-657
21. Beltrami AP, Barlucchi L, Torella D et al (2003) Adult cardiac stem cells are multipotent and support myocardial regeneration. Cell 114:763-776
22. Orlic D, Kajstura J, Chimenti S et al (2001) Bone marrow cells regenerate infarcted myocardium. Nature 410:701-705
23. Balsam LB, Wagers AJ, Christensen JL et al (2004) Haematopoietic stem cells adopt mature haematopoietic fates in ischaemic myocardium. Nature 428:668-673
24. Anversa P, Kajstura J, Leri A, Bolli R (2006) Life and death of cardiac stem cells: a paradigm shift in cardiac biology. Circulation 113:1451-1463
25. Yoon YS, Wecker A, Heyd L et al (2005) Clonally expanded novel multipotent stem cells from human bone marrow regenerate myocardium after myocardial infarction. J Clin Invest 115:326-338
26. Chen SL, Fang WW, Ye F et al (2004) Effect on left ventricular function of intracoronary transplantation of autologous bone marrow mesenchymal stem cell in patients with acute myocardial infarction. Am J Cardiol 94:92-95
27. Hare JM, Traverse JH, Henry TD et al (2009) A randomized, double-blind, placebo-controlled, dose-escalation study of intravenous adult human mesenchymal stem cells (prochymal) after acute myocardial infarction. J Am Coll Cardiol 54:2277-2286
28. Di Felice V, Zummo G (2009) Tetralogy of fallot as a model to study cardiac progenitor cell migration and differentiation during heart development. Trends Cardiovasc Med 19:130-135
29. Yerebakan C, Sandica E, Prietz S et al (2009) Autologous umbilical cord blood mononuclear cell transplantation preserves right ventricular function in a novel model of chronic right ventricular volume overload. Cell Transplant 18:855-868
30. Lombardi R, Marian AJ (2010) Arrhythmogenic right ventricular cardiomyopathy is a disease of cardiac stem cells. Curr Opin Cardiol [Epub ahead of print]

31. Ai D, Fu X, Wang J et al (2007) Canonical Wnt signaling functions in second heart field to promote right ventricular growth. Proc Natl Acad Sci U S A 104:9319-9324
32. D'Amario D, Fiorini C, Campbell PM et al (2011) Functionally competent cardiac stem cells can be isolated from endomyocardial biopsies of patients with advanced cardiomyopathies. Circ Res 108:857-861

Pathophysiology in Tetralogy of Fallot

5

Gabriele Egidy Assenza and Michael J. Landzberg

5.1 Introduction

Nowhere else in adult medicine does the world of congenital heart disease interdigitate so well with acquired heart disease as in the management of adult survivors of Tetralogy of Fallot (ToF). Progressive clinical dysfunction due to the combination of valvular pathology, abnormal loading conditions, maladaptive myocardial performance and abnormal interventricular and ventricular-arterial coupling can give the keen observer insights that have application throughout the wider cardiovascular practice.

This chapter serves as a basis for a better understanding of the pathology that affects the right ventricle in adults with repaired ToF. An extensive review of cardiac embryology appropriate to the student of the right ventricle and of ToF is followed by pathologic anatomy of the syndrome, and nature of modern surgical repair, all with an emphasis on the potential for development of right ventricular remodeling. The final sections discuss clinical study of right ventricular myocardial dysfunction in repaired ToF, and the rationale behind current investigative strategies designed to limit incapacity, and to improve outcomes.

5.2 Embryology of the Right Ventricle

The development of the human heart begins with the formation of the meso-dermic plate at the time of gastrulation during the third week of embryonic

M.J. Landzberg (✉)
Boston Adult Congenital Heart and Pulmonary Hypertension Program, Children's Hospital
Boston, Brigham and Women's Hospital, Harvard Medical School, Boston, MA, USA
e-mail: mike.landzberg@cardio.chboston.org

M. Chessa, A. Giamberti (eds.), *The Right Ventricle in Adults with Tetralogy of Fallot*,
© Springer-Verlag Italia 2012

Fig. 5.1 Components of the developing heart. *In green* are the venous tributaries and the distal aortic sac, while *purple* denotes the myocardium of the primary heart tube. The apical parts of the ventricles balloon in series from the primary tube, with the apical part of the left ventricle growing from the inlet components and the apical part of the right ventricle from the outlet component. *AVC*, Atrioventricular canal (from Moorman et al. [1], with permission)

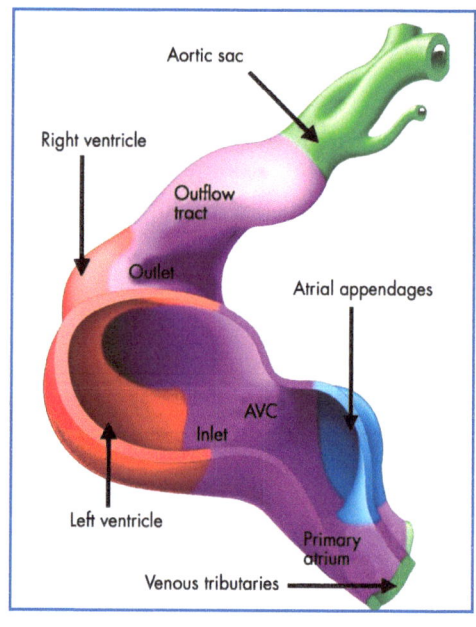

life. The mesodermic-derived cardiac precursors rapidly organize themselves in a tubular structure (the straight heart tube) which, due to the fold of the embryonic disk, is completely surrounded by the newly formed pericardial cavity [1]. At this stage the developing heart is centrally positioned within the embryo in a shape resembling an inverted Y (Fig. 5.1).

The two arms of this Y are caudal and are in continuity with the developing venous tributaries. This primary heart tube contains only the left ventricular precursor and part of the atria. The distal segment of the heart tube, which will be involved in right ventricular embryogenesis, is rapidly populated by a group of cells coming from a second cardiogenic area, located posterior to the dorsal wall of the developing pericardial cavity (the secondary heart field) [2]. Virtually all of the myocardium of the right ventricle and the myocardial lining of the outflow tract are from the secondary heart field. Proliferation, differentiation and addition of these cells to the heart tube depend on precise control of a number of transcription factors, including fibroblast growth factor 8 (FGF8) and T-box transcription factor 1 (TBX1). The importance of the secondary heart field in the normal embryogenesis of the cardiac outflow tract and right ventricle is emphasized in our current mechanistic understanding of DiGeorge syndrome, which is associated with conotruncal congenital cardiac abnormalities (including ToF, truncus arteriosus and interrupted aortic arch). Most individuals with DiGeorge syndrome possess a 1.5–3.0 Mb heterozygous 22q11.2 deletion which normally includes the region of *TBX1*, which is selectively expressed and functionally integrated in the pharyngeal mesenchyme cells of the secondary heart field [3].

Caudal and cranial additions to the straight tube produce elongation of the primary cardiac structure leading to a bend of the tube itself (looping of the heart tube). This looping is highly regulated by a complex signaling pathway, which involves numerous genes such as *lefty, nodal* and *Pitx2*. The bend is invariably rightward (dextro-looping) and brings the proximal (and caudal) portion of the Y-stem to be located to the left of the distal and cranial portion of the heart tube which is continued by the forming truncus arteriosus (outflow tract) (Fig. 5.1).

At this stage, all the blood from the atrial (venous) segment of the heart tube is required to pass through the entire ventricular looping to reach the outflow tract. As the tube bends, the primary interventricular foramen becomes obvious and delineates the boundary between the proximal and left-sided primitive ventricle (which will develop into the left ventricle) and the distal and right-sided bulbus cordis (which will develop as the right ventricle). After the looping, the tube itself has an inner and outer curvature and pronounced changes occur at both of these curvatures. The apical component of the right ventricle originates from the ballooning of the distal portion of the ventricular looping while the apical portion of the left ventricle is derived from the proximal outer curvature of the looping [4]. Interestingly, the timing of left and right ventricular myocardium formation is different; left ventricular myocardium is present even before looping of the heart tube, whereas right ventricular myocardium appears subsequently, ballooning out from the outlet limb of the primary tube [1].

Initially the solitary outflow tract of the straight heart tube is entirely aligned with the bulbus cordis (the future right ventricle), which initially supports both developing outflow tracts. During the last phase of cardiac embryogenesis, successful primary and secondary septation of the outflow tract allows walling the sub-aortic segment of the aortic sac with the newly formed left ventricle. Septation of the outflow depends on formation of the outflow ridges or cushions, which will create the so-called outflow septum (infundibular or conal septum). Usually, a pair of endocardial cushions develops in the solitary outflow tract. These cushions spiral around one another as they run from the distal end of the right ventricle to the aortic sac [2, 5]. They are populated by endocardial cells which undergo epithelial-mesenchymal transformation, originating from the secondary heart field cells and neural crest cells. The cardiac neural crest cells derive from the neural plate junction from the otic placode to the 4th somite and migrate via well-defined paths to reach first the pharyngeal apparatus and then the outflow ridges. Neural crest cells are instrumental in fusion of the ridges to form the outflow septum as well as for remodeling of the aortic arch system (which provides a framework to understand the co-segregation of conotruncal abnormalities with abnormalities of the aortic arch, such as the right aortic arch or interrupted aortic arch).

The outflow septum spirals as it passes from the pericardial reflection of the outflow tract toward the ventricles because of rotation of the myocardium of the proximal outflow – the part below the developing semilunar valves.

Inadequate or improper rotation of the proximal outflow tract results in what are often called conotruncal anomalies, including ToF, truncus arteriosus, transposition of the great arteries and double-outlet right ventricle. The myocardial cells in the walls of the proximal outflow tract grow into the proximal segment of the endocardial cushion, allowing a muscular partition of the outflow tract. This septum fuses and muscularizes. The progressive growth of this structure reduces the space beneath the free proximal edge of the fused outflow tract cushions. Eventually the entire leading edge of the fused outflow cushion becomes continuous with the right ventricular surface of the crest of the muscular ventricular septum, allowing the aorta to be connected to the left ventricular cavity and the pulmonary outflow to be in continuity with the right ventricle. Proper rotation of the outflow and development of the outflow septum result in two separate arterial roots aligned with their appropriate ventricle, along with closure of the interventricular foramen by the muscularized outflow septum as it joins the septal band (which is a muscle bundle running on the right surface of ventricular septum with two distinct limbs toward the right ventricular outflow tract) between its two limbs and the fused atrio-ventricular cushions.

Finally, the myocardium beneath the aorta (the subaortic conus) involutes, while the subpulmonary conus continues growing. This results in an expanded free-standing subpulmonary infundibulum above the right ventricle and mitral-to-aortic fibrous continuity on the left side. ToF appears to develop from improper junction of the outlet septum with the septal band and atrio-ventricular cushions. The outflow septum joins the left and superior limb of the septal band instead of the septal band, leaving the typical ventricular septal defect. The subpulmonary infundibulum fails to undergo normal expansion. The poorly expanded infundibulum, together with the displaced outlet septum results in pulmonary stenosis and an overriding aorta.

5.3   Right Ventricle in Tetralogy of Fallot: Anatomic Features

The right ventricle includes three recognized components (Fig. 5.2). The inflow (or inlet) portion runs from the tricuspid valve annulus to the attachment of the tensor apparatus of the tricuspid valve. The apical trabecular portion is between the inlet portion and the proximal os infundibuli. The proximal os infundibuli is identified by the septal band, the parietal band (which runs on the right ventricular free wall) and the moderator band, which connects the right ventricular free wall with the septal band. Distal to this muscular boundary, the os extends into the outflow (or outlet) portion of the right ventricle. The outflow portion of the right ventricle is defined proximally by the proximal os infundibuli and distally from the pulmonary valve annulus.

The septal bend presents a Y-shaped morphology, with the stem of the Y located toward the right ventricular apex. Toward the outflow tract, it is fused with the conal (infundibular) segment of the ventricular septum, which lies in

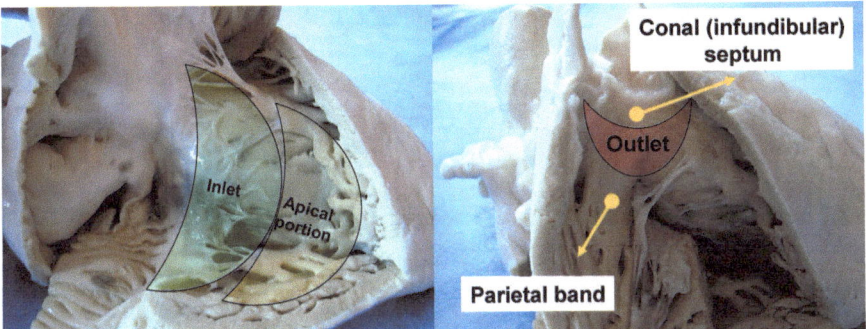

Fig. 5.2 Formalin-fixed specimen of a structurally normal heart. Right ventricular view showing the three components of the normal right ventricle. Courtesy of Dr. S. P. Sanders and Dr. F. Pluchinotta, Cardiac Registry, Children's Hospital Boston

the space between the two limbs of the Y. This spatial arrangement brings the conal septum so that it is located between the aortic and pulmonary valve.

Although ToF presents a wide morphologic spectrum, the classic four anatomic features which define the disease are all related to a single anatomic abnormality: the anterior, leftward and superior displacement of the conal septum. This anomaly variably narrows the right ventricular outflow tract, leading to subpulmonic obstruction. In addition, the displacement of this septum away from the posterior limb of the septal bend results in the typical malalignment type of ventricular septal defect. The aortic wall is immediately behind the conal septum so that the malaligned ventricular septal defect is always over-ridden by the left ventricular outflow tract, leading to unguarded right-to-left shunting (Fig. 5.3) [6]. Right ventricular hypertrophy is a consequence of right ventricular outflow tract obstruction and the systolic pressure equalization across the two ventricles due to the unrestrictive ventricular septal defect. The degree and distribution of right ventricular hypertrophy plays a fundamental role in the development of additional subpulmonary obstruction, since the hypertrophic anterior limb of the septal band and the septomarginal trabecula-tions (which are muscular bundles extending from the free right ventricular outflow tract wall) may contribute to muscular obstruction (which may need to be divided at the time of corrective surgery). In addition, in some instances, hypertrophy of the moderator band and apical trabeculations produces steno-sis at the level of the proximal os infundibuli, as seen in double chambered-right ventricle.

The atrioventricular node is normally located at the apex of Koch's triangle in patients with ToF [7]. In the majority of cases in which there is a malalign-ment type of ventricular septal defect, the bundle of His runs on the posterior and inferior rim of the defect, allowing ventricular septal defect closure with-out injury of the His bundle. Conversely, the right bundle branch runs very close to the ventricular septal defect and can be easily damaged at the time of

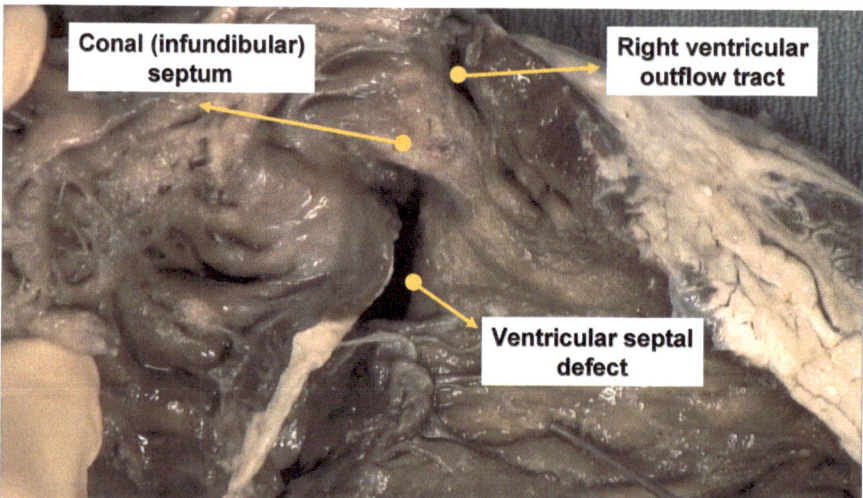

Fig. 5.3 Formalin-fixed specimen of a heart with ToF. The anteriorly and leftward displacement of the conal septum is shown along with the malilgnment ventricular septal defect and the narrow and obstructed right ventricular outflow tract. Note the severe degree of right ventricular hypertrophy. Courtesy of Dr. S. P. Sanders and Dr. F. Pluchinotta, Cardiac Registry, Children's Hospital Boston

surgical patch correction. This contributes to the high rate of complete right bundle branch block present in patients with repaired ToF (right ventricular conduction abnormality is also related to the presence of direct right ventriculotomy, as discussed in the next section). The conduction system never runs along the conal septum or the septomarginal trabeculation, which can be safely resected without the risk of producing heart block.

Patients with ToF experience long-term effects of chronic pressure and volume right ventricular overload. As discussed in the next section, the surgical repair of ToF causes a transition from severe pressure overload (when there is an unrepaired lesion with right ventricular outflow tract obstruction and unrestrictive ventricular septal defect and systolic ventricular pressure equalization) to chronic volume overload due to the effect of pulmonary valve disruption at the time of transannular patch plasty of the right ventricular outflow tract, leading to residual free pulmonary regurgitation. Interestingly, the three components of the right ventricle seem to be differentially affected by the long-term hemodynamic loading imposed by the pressure and volume overload. Cardiac magnetic resonance studies suggest that the apical trabecular portion of the right ventricle sustains the majority of the right ventricular remodeling and provides the largest contribution to stroke momentum of the right ventricle after ToF repair [8].

Right ventricular failure with cavity dilation, systolic dysfunction, myocardial fibrosis, leading to volume retention and symptoms of congestive heart failure are reported in the growing population of adults surviving with repaired ToF.

Although there are considerable data on the molecular events underlying left ventricular remodeling in a variety of human cardiac diseases, there is little information on the mechanism responsible for maladaptive remodeling of the overloaded right ventricle. Limited evidence suggests that those mechanisms could be different from the well established pathway described for the failing left ventricle. In one such example, limited study of renin-angiotensin system inhibition seems to suggest reduced benefit in patients with failing right ventricle in the context of complex congenital heart disease [9–10].

Animal models of pressure-loaded right ventricle (after pulmonary artery banding) suggest that right ventricular dilation and systolic dysfunction is coupled with increased cardiomyocyte apoptosis and extensive myocardial fibrosis [11]. Further studies have elucidated that chronic pressure overload is associated with abnormal and detrimental left ventricle to right ventricle interaction with abnormal septal motion, which leads to impaired diastolic filling of the left ventricle. In addition, limited evidence suggests that the presence of severe pressure loading on the right ventricle induces chamber-specific gene reprogramming, which seems to be distinct from what has been observed in animal models of left ventricular pressure overload [12]. This suggests that, in the context of acute and chronic right ventricular failure, a specific and orchestrated group of genes and gene-products may be up- or down-regulated. Such gene reprogramming could have a major impact on the specific phenotypic expression of right ventricular failure and could represent potential therapeutic targets to improve the overall prognosis of patients with failing right ventricle.

Dissecting the potential difference between left and right ventricular myocardium, mounting evidence suggests that the ability of right ventricular myocardium to adapt to chronic hypoxia is impaired in patients with ToF. The left ventricle presents several mechanisms to accommodate for severe hypoxia through the hypoxia-induced-factor (HIF)-1 pathway. These mechanisms include increased erythropoiesis and vascular endothelial growth factor-mediated angiogenesis, increase in glycolytic enzymes and sustained antioxidant activity through the glutathione-peroxidase activity, which has a protective effect on reperfusion injury. The right ventricular myocardium presents a hampered response to hypoxia. Real-time polymerase chain reaction data show that lower expression of the genes typically up-regulated in chronically hypoxic left ventricular myocardium is present in right ventricular myocardial samples from patients with ToF before the cyanotic phase prior to complete repair [13]. The implications of such early maladaptive response on long-term right ventricular function are currently unknown, but provide a framework to better understand long-term right ventricular myocardial failure in patients with cyanotic heart disease.

5.4   Complete Repair of Tetralogy of Fallot: Surgical Manipulation of the Right Ventricle

The goal of surgical intracardiac repair of ToF includes ventricular septal defect closure and complete relief of right ventricular outflow tract obstruction, allowing an optimal right-to-left ventricular pressure ratio post-operatively. Both goals require extensive surgical manipulation of either right ventricular outflow tract or ventricular septum and are associated with various degrees of surgical sequelae. Historically, very generous right ventriculotomy was performed so as to obtain excellent exposure of the intracardiac anatomy. This was associated with placement of a large transannular patch to obtain complete unobstructed right ventricular outflow tract. Although this surgical approach has the benefit of low incidence of residual outflow obstruction, it is invariably complicated by the development of free, or severe, pulmonary regurgitation, with the negative effect of chronic severe right ventricular volume overload, contributing to development of right ventricular dilation and dysfunction, exercise intolerance, congestive heart failure and increased cardiac mortality. In addition, the presence of such a large surgical incision on the free wall of the right ventricle acts as a hot spot for circuit reentry; this has been associated with increased risk of ventricular tachycardia and sudden death. Currently, when possible, access to the ventricular septal defect and the obstructing muscle bundle is achieved by an incision in either the right atrium or a combined incision also involving the pulmonary artery [6]. Right ventricular infundibulotomy is avoided when possible, and, when considered, is usually performed with a limited extension; this refinement of surgical technique has become increasingly popular as mild or modest residual right ventricular outflow tract gradient has been demonstrated not to be associated with worse peri-operative outcome (and often regresses within days after surgery). Closure of the ventricular septal defect is usually performed using patch material such as polytetrafluoroethylene (PTFE) or stretch-knitted Dacron [6]. Interrupted pledgeted polypropylene sutures may be used to sew the patch in place. Several critical anatomic points have to be sutured to avoid residual defects. If the septal band is not well developed, suturing of the posterior limb of the patch usually involves the septal leaflet of the tricuspid valve, which, at times, can distort the valve, leading to later development of tricuspid regurgitation.

The surgical handling of the complex right ventricular outflow tract obstruction requires resection of muscle bundles and the possible need for a transannular patch if the pulmonary valve is diminutive. To avoid the deleterious effect of severe pulmonary regurgitation, efforts are made to limit the disruption of the pulmonary valve. After valvar probing (using transatrial or right ventriculotomy approach) a longitudinal incision is made in the pulmonary artery. A full commisurotomy is performed (the valve is often bicuspid) and, afterwards, if the valve remains diminutive, a transannular incision is considered, with subsequent patch enlargement [6].

5.5 Adults with Tetralogy of Fallot: Does the Right Ventricle Influence the Natural History?

Right ventricular function and adaptation to adverse loading conditions in adults after repair of ToF has been the focus of a growing body of investigation in the last decade. Different factors can affect long-term right ventricular performance in this patient population and a wide range of right ventricular remodeling is observed in the adult population of patients late after ToF repair (Fig. 5.4). In addition to poor myocardial preservation at the time of initial repair, large ventriculotomy and chronic cyanosis before the repair, patients with corrected ToF face the unfavorable loading imposed by chronic pulmonary and tricuspid regurgitation, progressive myocardial fibrosis and scar, right and left ventricular dyssynchrony, multiple cardiopulmonary bypass runs and right ventricular pressure overload. Severe pulmonary regurgitation has been demonstrated to serve both as a mechanism for right ventricular dilation and dysfunction, as well as a risk factor for increased mortality. Establishing the link, however, between the progression of right ventricular dysfunction and

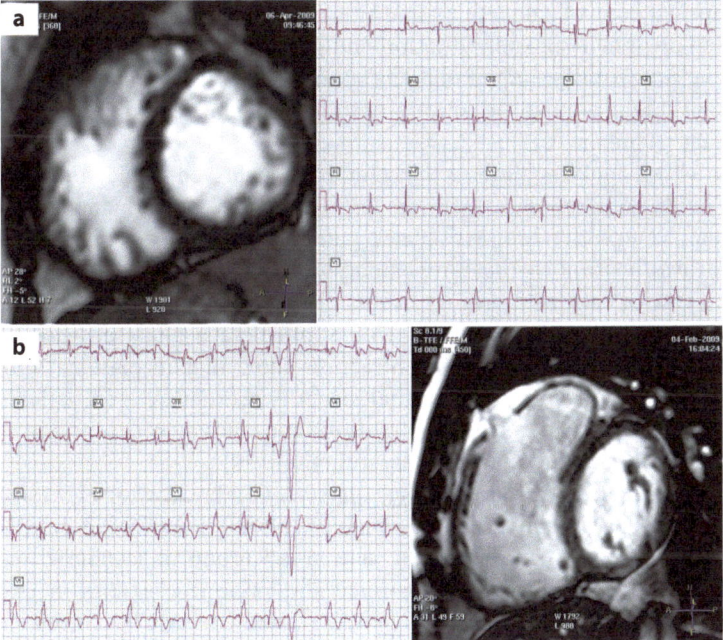

Fig. 5.4 Spectrum of disease. Cardiac magnetic resonance still frame from a steady-state free precession cine imaging in diastole, in a short axis view, coupled with respective electrocardiogram in two patients with repaired ToF. The comparison between **a** and **b** exemplifies the wide range of right ventricular dimension affecting QRS duration seen in adults with repaired ToF. Courtesy of Dr. A. J. Powell, Cardiac Magnetic Resonance Program, Children's Hospital Boston

the hard clinical endpoints of exercise intolerance, congestive heart failure and increased cardiac mortality remains a challenge for investigators. Since pulmonary valve replacement is an available option to correct this abnormality, a large body of medical study is trying to define the benefits and optimal timing of such intervention, trading off the increased right ventricular preservation with the risk and consequences of this surgical procedures. Multiple retrospective studies tried to define the benefit of pulmonary valve replacement to promote right ventricular remodeling after surgery, decrease the arrhythmic burden, improve exercise tolerance and reduce cardiac outcomes [14–16]. Although pulmonary valve replacement appears to be a reasonable option in patients with the most severe pulmonary regurgitation and dysfunctional right ventricles, symptoms and a higher degree of arrhythmic burden, the exact timing of the operation and the overall effect on natural history of these patients remains to be further elucidated [17].

The mechanics of right ventricular contraction in patients with repaired ToF has been extensively studied with innovative approaches such as cardiac magnetic resonance and speckle-tracking echocardiography. Those investigations have revealed that even in the presence of relatively preserved right ventricular function, a delayed activation of the right ventricular outflow tract is present in persons with repaired ToF as compared to that observed in right ventricles from normal control subjects. In addition, such delays seem to correlate with the degree of right ventricular dilation and pulmonary regurgitation, suggesting that the unfavorable sequential activation of the right ventricle could be associated or might predispose to long-term detrimental remodeling of the right ventricular chamber.

Speckle-tracking analysis showed that abnormal right ventricular function is associated with unfavorable effects on left ventricular performance. This concept of inter-ventricular interaction has gained increasing acceptance as left ventricular dysfunction has been repeatedly demonstrated to be associated with increased risk of cardiac mortality in this disease, as well as in other primary pathologies of the right ventricle [18]. Sophisticated analyses such as longitudinal strain of left ventricular contraction show that in patients with ToF a depressed left ventricular myocardial strain is present even in patients with preserved left ventricular ejection fraction, and that such depression is related to the degree of right ventricular dysfunction [19].

Late right ventricular dysfunction has also been related to progressive myocardial fibrosis. Cardiac magnetic resonance with intravenous gadolinium administration has been extensively used in a broad group of ischemic and non-ischemic cardiomyopathies to investigate the presence, extension and relation of myocardial fibrosis to ventricular function, exercise performance and functional status, and survival outcomes in non- congenital heart disease. More recently, late gadolinium enhancement has been used to study patients with complex heart disease and systemic right ventricle as well as in patients with repaired ToF [20–21]. Although the presence of abnormal late gadolinium enhancement is very common in adults with repaired ToF (in particular in specific locations of surgical manipulation such as the right ventricular out-flow tract or the ventricular septal patch), the extension of delayed right ventricular myocardial enhancement has been related to increased arrhythmic burden, global right ventricular dysfunction and exercise intolerance. Myocardial fibrosis could result from early myocardial injury at the time of the initial repair or could represent the final common pathway of a maladaptive response to chronic insult. Interestingly, age and age at repair both seem to correlate with higher extension of abnormal enhancement, suggesting that more aggressive right ventricular manipulation, poor myocardial preservation and ongoing insult could be responsible for such injury. In addition the extent of regional delayed enhancement in the right ventricular outflow tract has been associated with global right ventricular dysfunction and poor exercise capacity [22].

The abnormal mechanical activation of the right ventricle has been studied using biomedical engineering techniques involving concepts such as stroke work and energy transfer. Comparing right ventricles from normal control subjects to those from persons with repaired ToF, higher operating pressure with lower computed stroke work and higher negative energy transfer at the level of pulmonary artery has been shown in the population with congenital heart disease [23]. These investigations suggest that the right ventricle in ToF presents a less efficient profile compared to normal anatomy.

The significance and progressive nature of right ventricular dysfunction has prompted study of potential clinical strategies that can limit the ongoing insult to the right ventricle, reducing the hemodynamic burden and improving long-term biventricular performance. Translating this information on right ventricular performance and myocardial abnormality into a clinical model able to predict the impact of such derangements on the natural history of this patient population is one of the major goals of clinical research in adult congenital heart disease. Survival after ToF repair greatly exceeds past expectations, with yearly incidence of major cardiac outcomes (such as sudden death, sustained ventricular tachycardia or refractory congestive heart failure requiring advanced mechanical support or heart transplantation) being low. However, the occurrence of these outcomes greatly increases with the age of the population. Given a significant change in slope of occurrence of adversity with increasing decades of subject age, retrospective studies looking at outcome prediction face the challenge of both the need for very long follow-up as well as the constraints of small individual institutional population cohort size. Limited data suggest that right ventricular performance does impact on functional capacity and major adverse outcomes late after ToF repair [24, 25]. Recently, an international, multicenter registry has been established to help define risk factors for late adverse outcomes in adults with ToF [26]. The goal of this approach, combining data collection regarding muscle function and clinical outcomes from multiple institutions with large patient cohorts, is to overcome the existing limitations and to provide both stronger clinical evidence and rationale behind strategies to sustain right ventricular health and to thereby improve long-term outcome for adults surviving long after the repair of ToF.

References

1. Moorman A, Webb S, Brown NA et al (2003) Development of the heart: (1) formation of the cardiac chambers and arterial trunks. Heart 89:806-814
2. Waldo KL, Kumiski DH, Wallis KT et al (2001) Conotruncal myocardium arises from a secondary heart field. Development 128:3179-3188
3. Nowotschin S, Liao J, Gage PJ et al (2006) Tbx1 affects asymmetric cardiac morphogenesis by regulating Pitx2 in the secondary heart field. Development 133:1565-1573
4. Lamers WH, Moorman AF (2002) Cardiac septation: a late contribution of the embryonic primary myocardium to heart morphogenesis. Circ Res 91:93-103
5. Anderson RH, Webb S, Brown NA et al (2003) Development of the heart: (3) formation of the ventricular outflow tracts, arterial valves, and intrapericardial arterial trunks. Heart 89:1110-1118
6. Duncan BW (2010) Tetralogy of Fallot with Pulmonary stenosis. In: Sellke, FW, del Nido PJ, Swanson SJ (eds) Surgery of the Chest. Saunders, Elsevier, Philadelphia, pp 1877-1896
7. Gatzoulis MA, Babu-Narayan SV (2011) Tetralogy of Fallot. In: Gatzoulis MD, Webb GD, Daubeney PEF (eds) Diagnosis and management of adult congenital heart disease: Saunders, Elsevier, Philadelphia, pp 316-327
8. Bodhey NK, Beerbaum P, Sarikouch S et al (2008) Functional analysis of the components of the right ventricle in the setting of tetralogy of Fallot. Circ Cardiovasc Imaging 1:141-147
9. Dore A, Houde C, Chan KL et al (2005) Angiotensin receptor blockade and exercise capacity in adults with systemic right ventricles: a multicenter, randomized, placebo-controlled clinical trial. Circulation 112:2411-2416
10. Babu-Narayan SV, Uebing A, Davlouros PA et al (2010) Randomised trial of ramipril in repaired tetralogy of Fallot and pulmonary regurgitation The APPROPRIATE study (Ace inhibitors for Potential PRevention Of the deleterious effects of Pulmonary Regurgitation In Adults with repaired TEtralogy of Fallot). Int J Cardiol [Epub ahead of print]
11. Minegishi S, Kitahori K, Murakami A et al (2011) Mechanism of pressure-overload right ventricular hypertrophy in infant rabbits. Int Heart J 52:56-60
12. Urashima T, Zhao M, Wagner R et al (2008) Molecular and physiological characterization of RV remodeling in a murine model of pulmonary stenosis. Am J Physiol Heart Circ Physiol 295:H1351-H1368
13. Reddy S, Osorio JC, Duque AM et al (2006) Failure of right ventricular adaptation in children with tetralogy of Fallot. Circulation 114:I37-I42
14. Oosterhof T, van Straten A, Vliegen HW et al (2007) Preoperative thresholds for pulmonary valve replacement in patients with corrected tetralogy of Fallot using cardiovascular magnetic resonance. Circulation 116:545-551
15. Frigiola A, Tsang V, Bull C et al (2008) Biventricular response after pulmonary valve replacement for right ventricular outflow tract dysfunction: is age a predictor of outcome? Circulation 118:S182-S190
16. Eyskens B, Reybrouck T, Bogaert J et al (2000) Homograft insertion for pulmonary regurgitation after repair of tetralogy of fallot improves cardiorespiratory exercise performance. Am J Cardiol 85:221-225
17. Harrild DM, Berul CI, Cecchin F et al (2009) Pulmonary valve replacement in tetralogy of Fallot: impact on survival and ventricular tachycardia. Circulation 119:445-451
18. Ghai A, Silversides C, Harris L et al (2002) Left ventricular dysfunction is a risk factor for sudden cardiac death in adults late after repair of tetralogy of Fallot. J Am Coll Cardiol 40:1675-1680
19. Kempny A, Diller GP, Orwat S et al (2010) Right ventricular-left ventricular interaction in adults with Tetralogy of Fallot: A combined cardiac magnetic resonance and echocardiographic speckle tracking study. Int J Cardiol [Epub ahead of print]
20. Babu-Narayan SV, Goktekin O, Moon JC et al (2005) Late gadolinium enhancement cardiovascular magnetic resonance of the systemic right ventricle in adults with previous atrial redirection surgery for transposition of the great arteries. Circulation 111:2091-2098

21. Babu-Narayan SV, Kilner PJ, Li W et al (2006) Ventricular fibrosis suggested by cardiovascular magnetic resonance in adults with repaired tetralogy of fallot and its relationship to adverse markers of clinical outcome. Circulation 113:405-413
22. Wald RM, Haber I, Wald R et al (2009) Effects of regional dysfunction and late gadolinium enhancement on global right ventricular function and exercise capacity in patients with repaired tetralogy of Fallot. Circulation 119:1370-1377
23. Das A, Banerjee RK, Gottliebson WM (2010) Right ventricular inefficiency in repaired tetralogy of Fallot: proof of concept for energy calculations from cardiac MRI data. Ann Biomed Eng 38:3674-3687
24. Lu JC, Cotts TB, Agarwal PP et al (2010) Relation of right ventricular dilation, age of repair, and restrictive right ventricular physiology with patient-reported quality of life in adolescents and adults with repaired tetralogy of fallot. Am J Cardiol 106:1798-1802
25. Knauth AL, Gauvreau K, Powell AJ et al (2008) Ventricular size and function assessed by cardiac MRI predict major adverse clinical outcomes late after tetralogy of Fallot repair. Heart 94:211-216
26. Valente AM, Babu-Narayan S, Assenza GE et al (2011) International multicenter tetralogy of Fallot registry: Identifying predictors of adverse outcomes using cardiac MRI parameters. Journal of Cardiovascular Magnetic Resonance Imaging 13:187

Tetralogy of Fallot: Late Outcome

Jochen Weil

6.1   Introduction

Tetralogy of Fallot (ToF) is the most frequent cyanotic congenital heart disease (CHD). According to a recent prospective study on the prevalence of CHD in Germany, 0.27 of 10,000 live born neonates (2.5% of all CHD) suffer from ToF [1].

Without treatment this frequently occurring CHD has a high morbidity and mortality. Surgical treatment has improved this grim outlook dramatically.

In the following chapter, the long-term survival and morbidity of the natural and unnatural history will be summarized.

6.2   Natural History

The degree of central cyanosis in patients with ToF depends on the severity of the right ventricular outflow tract obstruction (RVOTO). In early infancy the cyanosis might be less significant, but with increasing age the RVOTO becomes more severe and the patient more cyanotic.

Before the era of palliative or corrective surgery the mortality and morbidity of unoperated patients was high.

In 1978 E.G. Bertranou and coworkers [2] analyzed all published autopsy cases of patients with ToF who died without surgical treatment, in order to determine the life expectancy of such patients. These data were compared with a study of patients alive in Denmark in 1949 [3]. The rates of survival accord-

J. Weil (✉)

Department of Pediatric Cardiology, University Heart Center Hamburg,
Hamburg, Germany
e-mail: jweil@uke.de

M. Chessa, A. Giamberti (eds.), *The Right Ventricle in Adults with Tetralogy of Fallot,*
© Springer-Verlag Italia 2012

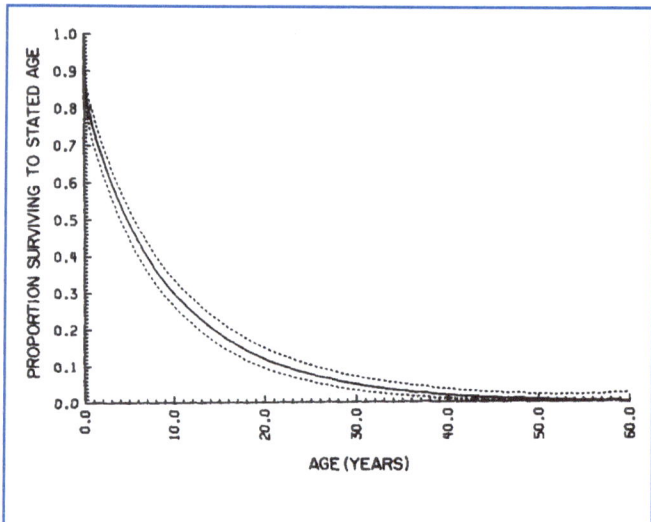

Fig. 6.1 Life expectancy of people with ToF without pulmonary atresia (from Bertranou et al. [2], with permission)

ing to these two sources were remarkably similar. According to this data, 75% of patients with ToF and pulmonary stenosis were alive at 1 year, 60% at 3 years and only 30% at 10 years of age (Fig. 6.1).

In the subset of patients with ToF and pulmonary atresia the survival rates were lower than in patients with pulmonary stenosis, indicating that only 66% of patients were alive at age 6 months, 50% at 1 year, 33% at 2 years and 8% at 18 years old.

These data were comparable to other publications. Samanek [4] studied the probability of survival in non-operated children with CHD in Bohemia. For the patients with ToF the actuarial survival rate at 1 year was 64%, at 5 years 49%, at 10 years 23% and only 4% at 15 years. Campbell [5] found the mean age of death in patients with ToF was 8.9 years.

There are several case reports of individuals with non treated ToF and unusual longevity, such as the report on the American composer Henry Gilbert who died 8 days following left hemiplegia within a few months of his 60th birthday [6].

Morbidity in adult survivors of ToF without surgery is high. The chronic hypoxemia results in exercise intolerance and excessive erythrocytosis with an increased risk of thrombosis. Cerebral abscesses are frequent since infectious agents can easily reach the brain via right to left shunting on a ventricular level. The risk of thrombosis and brain abscess is increased in the presence of iron deficiency due to the impaired rheology of the blood.

Death occurs frequently secondary to right ventricular (RV) failure due to long standing RV pressure load and secondary to endocarditis or to arrhythmias.

6.3 Patients with Repaired ToF

The introduction of surgical repair of ToF has dramatically improved survival and decreased the morbidity in these patients.

There are a number of issues that are important to consider for the long-term care of adult patients surviving surgical repair of ToF.

The following issues are dealt in this chapter:

- survival
- reoperations
- changes in the left heart.

The issues of pulmonary valve regurgitations with the requirement of pulmonary valve replacement, arrhythmia and sudden death are covered in their respective chapters.

6.3.1 Long-term Survival After Repair

It is obvious that the era in which a patient was operated influences the outcome, as well the age in which the patient underwent the repair.

Kirklin and coworkers [7] reported a hospital mortality of 50% in 1955 and 15% in 1960. Nowadays the hospital mortality will be less than 5% in patients after repair in most centers [8, 9].

There are several recent publications reporting excellent survival over 3 decades after successful staged or primary repair.

Murphy and co-workers [10] reviewed the records of all patients who underwent complete surgical repair of ToF at the Mayo Clinic (USA) between 1955 and 1960 and survived the immediate (30 days) postoperative period. The overall 32 years actuarial survival rate among 163 patients was 86% as compared with an expected rate of 96% in a control population matched for age and sex (Fig. 6.2).

The survival rates among patients less than 12 years of age at the time of repair ranged between 90 and 93%, which was slightly less than the expected rates. Among patients 12 years old or older at the time of surgery, however, the survival rate was only 76%, compared with an expected rate of 93%.

Primary palliation with a Blalock-Taussig shunt before repair was not associated with reduced long-term survival, nor was the need for a transannular patch at the time of surgery.

A systolic RV-left ventricular (LV) pressure ratio of 0.5 and greater was predictive of a higher mortality during the first 20 years after surgery (92% versus 88% after 20 years).

Most patients had a good functional status with 77% of patients in New York Heart Association (NYHA) functional class I, 17% in class II and 6% in class III at the late follow-up examination. Late sudden cardiac death occurred in ten patients.

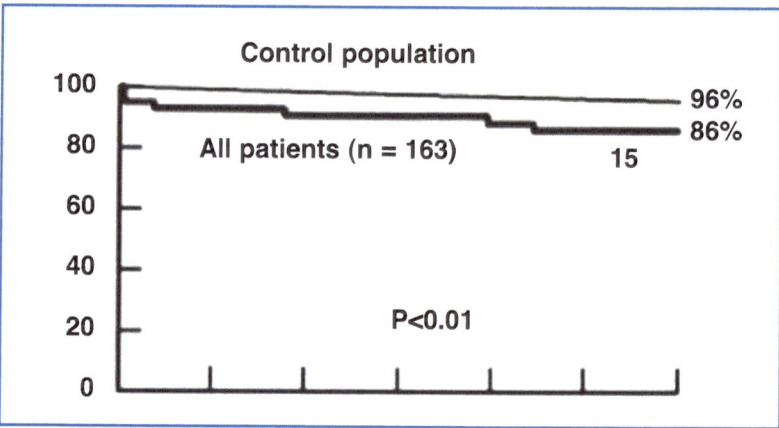

Fig. 6.2 Long-term survival of patients with complete repair of ToF who survived the immediate postoperative period. This panel shows the actuarial survival rate up to 32 years after surgery for all patient groups combined and the expected survival rate in an age- and sex-matched control population (from Murphy et al. [10], with permission)

This study provides evidence that the rate of long-term survival – even in the earliest era of opens heart surgery – is excellent, but remains lower than in the general population. The actuarial survival rate was 90% of the expected survival rate. The late functional status was also excellent. The occurrence of late sudden cardiac death accounted for approximately half of all late deaths.

Similar good long-term results were reported by Nollert and co-workers in 490 patients who were operated upon in Munich (Germany) from 1958 to 1977 and who survived the first year after surgical repair [11]. They found actuarial 10, 20, 30 and 36 year survival rates of 97%, 94%, 89% and 85%, respectively. The most common cause of death was sudden cardiac death (n=13) followed by congestive heart failure (n=6).

It is important to realize that mortality increased 25 years after surgery from 0.24% to 0.94% per year, emphasizing the need for close life-long follow-up examinations (Fig. 6.3).

In a single center's 50 year experience with surgical management of ToF, Lindberg and co-workers reported the long-term outcome in 570 patients showing that there was no difference in freedom from death or reoperation following primary repair versus primary palliation [8] (Fig. 6.4). This finding was in agreement with the previous publications by Nollert and co-workers [11].

Furthermore it was shown that there was no difference in long-term survival between patients with and without transannular patch [8, 9].

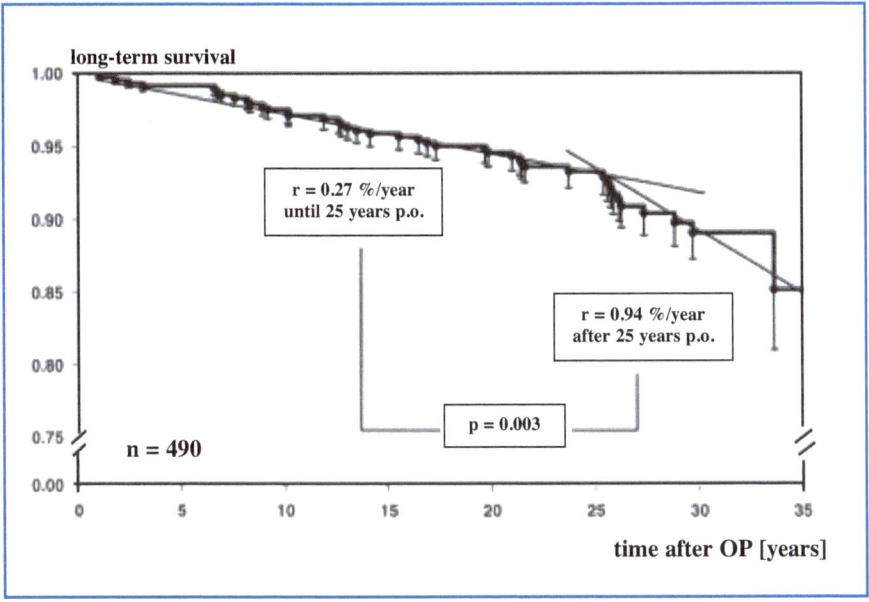

Fig. 6.3 Long-term survival after correction of ToF. All patients who died within the first year after correction were excluded from calculation of long-term survival. The curve shows two different phases that are distinct. The early, low first phase lasts 25 years; thereafter, the risk increases significantly. Mortality risk (r) per year, as a linearized number, is calculated for each phase. Note the break in the y axis. *OP*, operation; *p.o.*, postoperatively (from Nollert et al. [11], with permission)

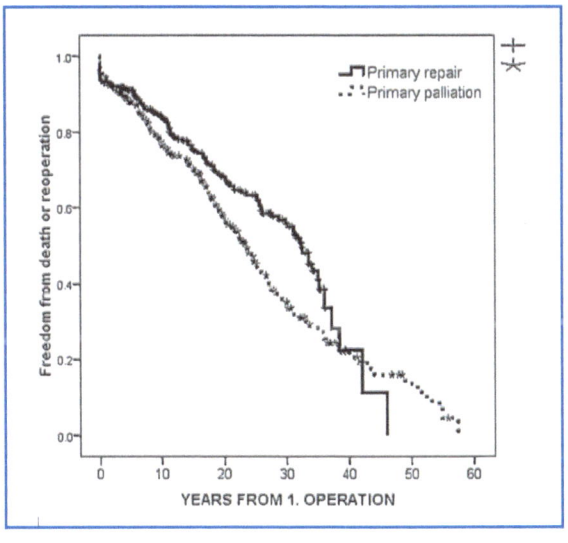

Fig. 6.4 Long-time follow-up after different approaches in surgical treatment of primary repair or primary palliative surgery (from Lindberg et al. [8], with permission)

6.3.2 Reoperations

As shown, the long-term survival of patients after repair for ToF is excellent. These patients, however, continue to be at risk for long-term morbidity. With increasing length of follow-up from the time of primary surgery, problems will occur such as:

- stenosis of the RVOT
- pulmonary valve regurgitation
- branch pulmonary arteries
- regurgitation of tricuspid valve.

These problems may be well tolerated in the early years after operation, but with longer periods of long-term follow-up they will result an increased risk of ventricular and supraventricular arrhythmia, heart failure and sudden cardiac death.

Reoperation is required in about 10–30% in patients with ToF during long-term follow-up [10, 12–14].

The group from the Toronto Congenital Cardiac Center for Adults reviewed its experience with reoperation in adults who got their primary repair at a mean age of 13.3 years [12]. Out of a total of 330 patients with repaired ToF over 18 years of age, 60 consecutive patients underwent reoperation between 1975 and 1997. Mean age at reoperation was 33.3 years and the mean follow-up after reoperation was 5 years.

The most common indication for reoperation was complications of the RVOT in 75% of patients. Severe pulmonary valve regurgitation (38%) and conduit failure (22%) were the most frequent problems of the RVOT. Less frequent indications were a significant leak after patch closure of the ventricular septal defect (VSD) and severe tricuspid valve regurgitation.

A bioprosthetic valve to reconstruct the RVOT was used in 42 out 60 patients.

According to this study the number of reoperations increased in the recent years. Within the last 6 years (1990–1996) 72% of all reoperations were performed (Fig. 6.5).

There was no perioperative mortality. The most recent follow-up examinations revealed excellent results after reoperation: 93% of the patients were in NYHA classification I or II. Actuarial 10 year survival reached 92% (Fig. 6.6).

In an earlier retrospective study from the Mayo Clinic (USA) a reoperation rate was found in 10% (16 patients) of 163 survivors who had their repair between 1955 and 1960 [10]. At that time the principal reasons for late reoperations were residual VSD (ten patients) and false aneurysm of the pulmonary outflow tract (three patients). Only two out of 16 patients requiring reoperations got a valve replacement for severe pulmonary valve insufficiency.

The use of a transannular patch does not influence the long-term survival, but increases the risk of reoperation due to severe pulmonary valve regurgitation.

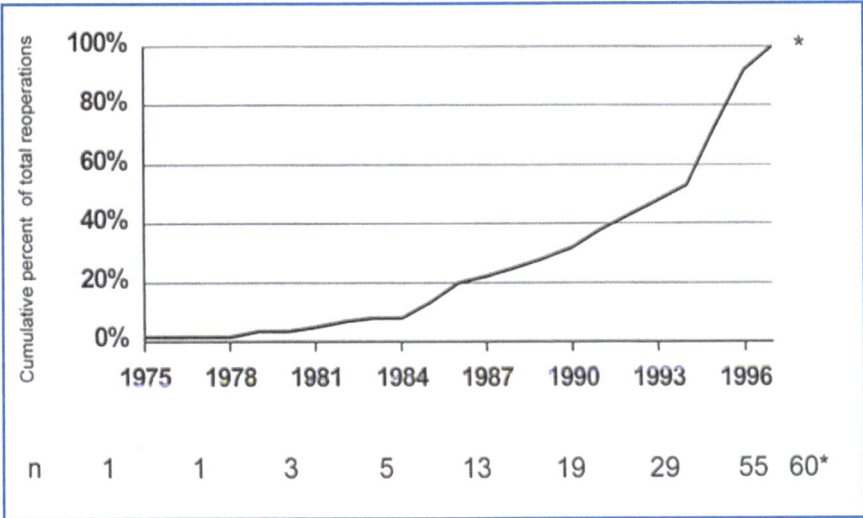

Fig. 6.5 Cumulative percent of reoperations from 1975 until March 1997. There is a marked increase of reoperations in recent years. *N*, numbers of reoperation; *, denotes March 31, 1997 (from Oechslin et al. [12], with permission)

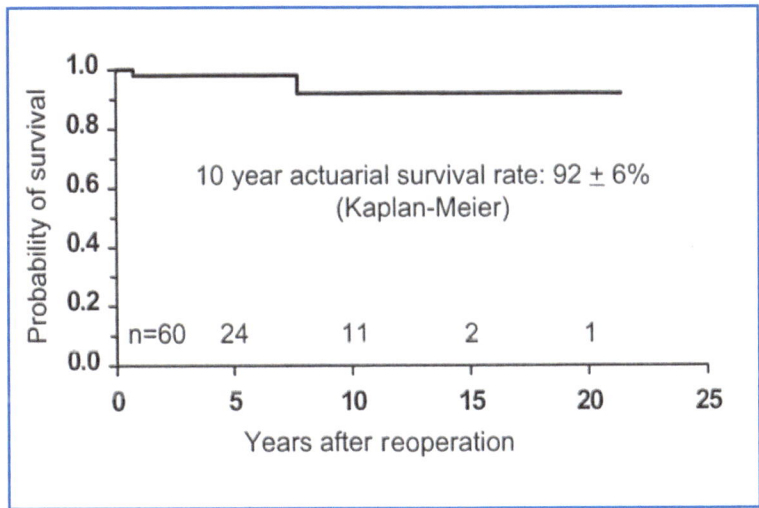

Fig. 6.6 Kaplan-Meier actuarial survival analysis for patients after reoperation. *N*, number of patients entering each time interval (from Oechslin et al. [12], with permission)

Fig. 6.7 The influence of repair crossing the pulmonary
annulus upon freedom from
reoperation following surgery for ToF (from Lind-
berg et al. [8], with permission)

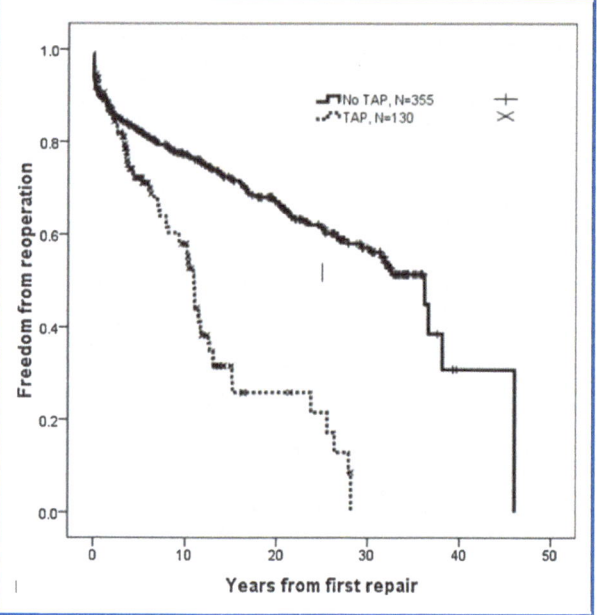

Lindberg and co-workers showed that freedom from reoperation was highly significantly reduced in patients repaired with a transannular patch compared to patients without such a repair [8] (Fig. 6.7). These authors did not find
an influence of previous palliation, transatrial or transventricular repair on the
rate of survival or reoperations.

Similar results were published by Park and co-workers [13]. They found a
rate of reoperation or intervention in 31, 7% (224 patients) of 734 patients.
The most common causes for reoperation or re-intervention were pulmonary
valve regurgitation in 109 patients and branch pulmonary artery stenosis in
127 patients. It was shown that preservation of the pulmonary annulus can
reduce the reoperation rate.

Interestingly the rate of reoperations seems not to have changed over the
last decades. The frequency of reoperations did not differ significantly during
five decades from 1959–2009, according to the publication by Lindberg and
co-workers [8] (Fig. 6.8).

It is anticipated that the rate and the mode of reoperations will change in
the present time or in the future.

Nowadays intraoperative echocardiography is performed in most centers.
With the help of this intraoperative monitoring of the surgical results, a residual VSD, significant tricuspid valve regurgitation or a severe RVOTO can be
detected and treated immediately. These lesions should require less frequent
reoperation than they did decades ago.

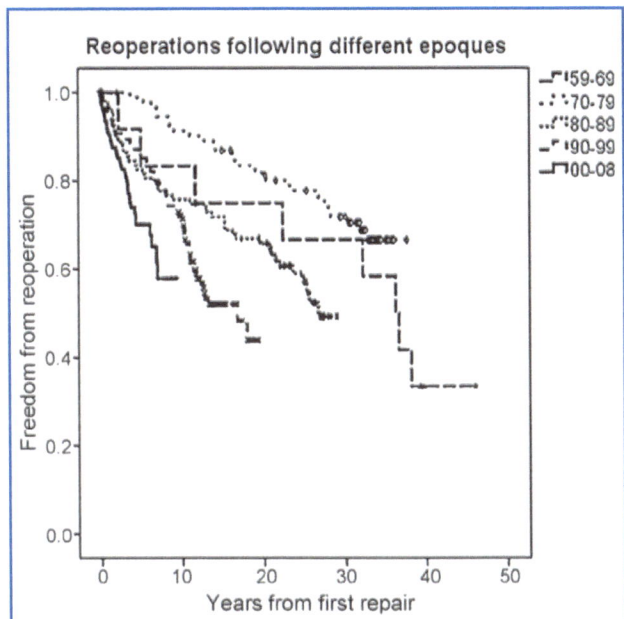

Fig. 6.8 Survival and frequency of reoperations during the five different decennials following surgery for ToF (from Lindberg et al. [8], with permission)

It is now well recognized that repair with a transannular patch will result in an increased late morbidity and need for reoperation due to severe pulmonary regurgitation. To avoid severe pulmonary regurgitation a residual gradient of the RVOT with a RV to LV pressure ratio of about 0.5 is accepted performing a surgical enlargement of the RVOT only up to -2 SD of normal.

Furthermore, many reoperations can be replaced by non-surgical treatment in the catheterization laboratory. The most common morbidity in the long-term outlook is a problem with the RVOT and the pulmonary arteries.

Stenosis of branch pulmonary arteries can be now treated in most patients with balloon dilatation and/or implantation of stents. Re-stenosis or insufficiency of a RV to pulmonary artery conduit are amenable to percutaneous pulmonary valve replacement (see chapters 10 and 11).

6.3.3 Right-left Ventricular Interaction

Despite an excellent long-term survival after repair of ToF, many patients show significant morbidity. This morbidity will increase with time after repair and is thought to be caused mainly by problems of the right heart such as stenosis and insufficiency of pulmonary valve with consecutive RV pressure and volume load. These changes lead to a reduced RV function with decreased exercise tolerance and functional status as well atrial and ventricular arrhythmia and sudden death.

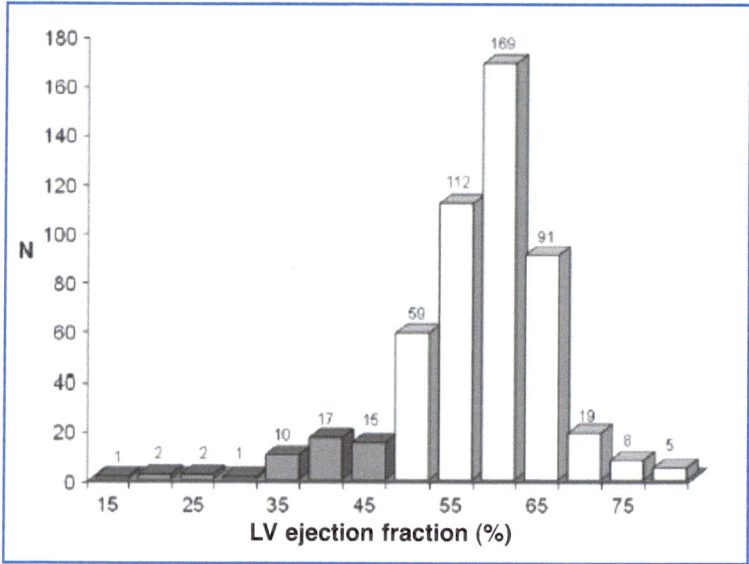

Fig. 6.9 Histogram of estimated left ventricular ejection fraction displays the lower limit of each category (*x-axis labels*) and decreased ejection fraction (*gray bars*) (from Broberg et al. [15], with permission)

Within the last years it has become obvious that the changes of the right heart after repair for ToF will affect the morphology and performance of the left heart. In patients with repaired ToF an important part of morbidity in long-term follow-up is caused by LV dysfunction and has to be considered for the management of these patients.

Broberg and co-workers studied the LV function with echocardiography in 511 adult patients with a mean age of 37.2 years [15]. All patients had a successful repair of ToF performed at a median age of 6 years. In this large cross-sectional study LV systolic dysfunction was found in 20,9% of patients with ToF. LV dysfunction was defined as a left ventricular ejection fraction (LVEF) less than 55%, showing increased LV diameter, decreased fractional LV shortening and a reduced myocardial performance index. A moderately (EF 35–44%) and severely (EF less than 35%) reduced LV function was found in 5,2% and 1,1%, respectively, out of the 20.9% of patients with LV dysfunction (Fig. 6.9).

There was a strong association between a reduced RV function and LV dysfunction. Most patients with normal LV function had normal RV function (67%). In patients with moderately to severe LV dysfunction, only 28% had a normal right ventricle, whereas 44% had a moderate to severe RV dysfunction (Fig. 6.10).

Interestingly, there was no relation between the severity of pulmonary regurgitation and LV function. This is in accordance with a study by Geva et al.

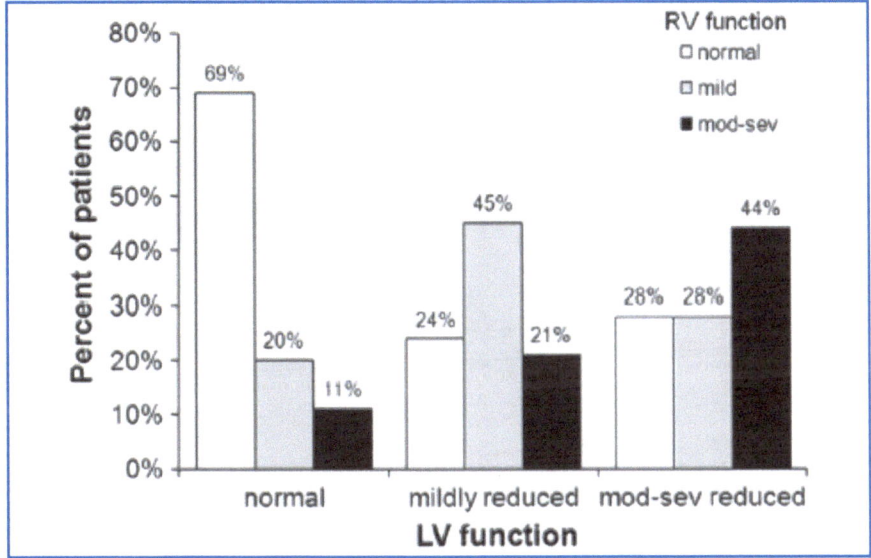

Fig. 6.10 Patients with normal right ventricular function were more likely to have normal left ventricular function. In contrast, moderate-severe (*mod-sev*) right ventricular dysfunction was more prevalent in patients with moderately to severely decreased left ventricular dysfunction (p <0.001, chi-square test) (from Broberg et al. [15], with permission)

[16], who did not find a correlation between the degree of pulmonary valve regurgitation and impaired clinical status.

A strong association, however, could be found between LV dysfunction and arrhythmia. Patients with LV dysfunction showed a wider QRS duration and more often had previous arrhythmia or implantation of a pacemaker and cardioverter-defibrillator, respectively.

The assumption that reduced LV function results in an increased risk of arrhythmia was supported by a retrospective survey of implanted cardioverter-defibrillator discharges in patients with ToF [17, 18]. In this study the strongest independent predictor for appropriate shock delivery was an increased LV end-diastolic pressure, more than RV dysfunction, QRS duration or syncope.

There is further evidence that there is a close relationship between reduced RV and LV dysfunction suggesting an unfavorable ventricular-ventricular interaction in patients with repaired ToF. Geva and co-workers studied 100 consecutive patients with a median age of 21 years after repair [16]. They correlated the clinical functional class of these patients with the ejection fraction of RV and LV determined by cardiac Magnetic Resonance Tomography (MRT). They found that a low LV ejection fraction – more than a RV-dysfunction – was the strongest independent factor associated with impaired clinical status. The combination of lower LVEF (less than 40%) and older age at ToF

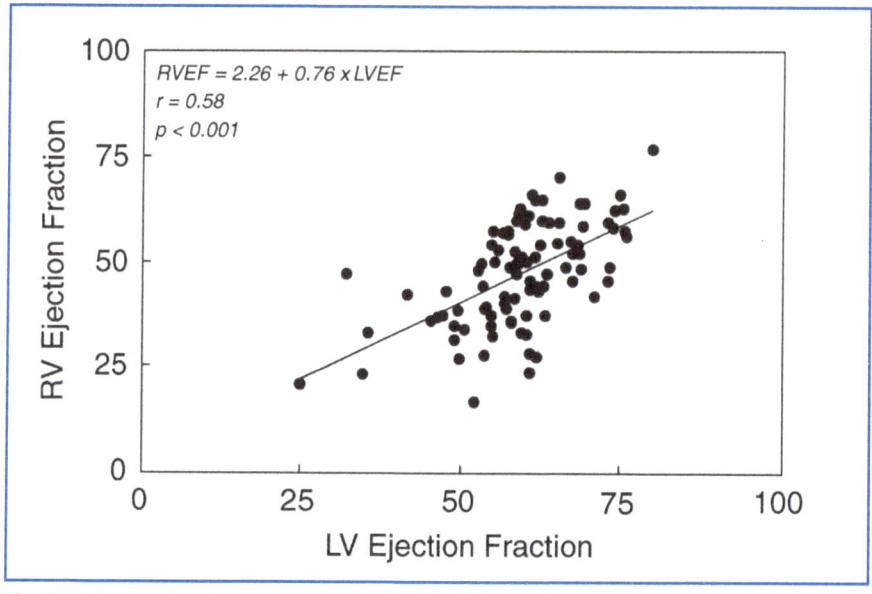

Fig. 6.11 Association between right ventricular (*RV*) and left ventricular (*LV*) ejection fraction (*EF*) (from Geva et al. [16], with permission)

repair had a high sensitivity and specificity for being in NYHA functional class greater than III.

Furthermore, a significant correlation was found between RV and LV ejection fraction in these patients (Fig. 6.11).

This finding confirmed the results of a previous publication in adults after ToF repair, which showed an adverse right-to-left ventricular interaction in patients with RVOT aneurysm or akinesia [19].

All these data underline the necessity not only of focusing on RV mechanics and their interaction with pulmonary valve regurgitation, but also on concomitant dysfunction of the LV. The mechanism that links RV dysfunction to a decrease in LV function is not clearly understood. Possible causes for LV dysfunction could be chronic hypoxemia, altered mechanics of interventricular septum due to patch closure of VSD and volume loading of RV, damage to coronary arteries during repair or altered electro-mechanical interactions due to a long QRS duration.

Another cause for ventricular dysfunction could be ventricular fibrosis. Babu-Narayan et al. [20] examined the extent of fibrosis in RV and LV detected by late gadolinium enhancement (LGE) using cardiovascular MRT in 92 adult patients with repaired ToF. Besides marked fibrosis in different parts of the RV they found LGE in the LV (53%) not only at the apex consistent with apical vent insertion (49%), but also in the inferior or lateral wall consistent with infarction (5%) or in other areas (8%) (Fig. 6.12).

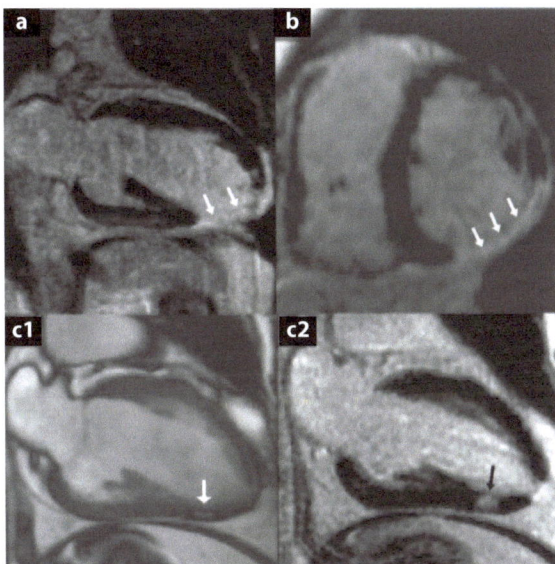

Fig. 6.12 Examples of LV LGE late after ToF repair. **a**, **b** Images illustrating unexpected LV infarction (*arrows*) in two different patients. **c** A further example of localized LV LGE in another patient. The cineframe in **c1** and corresponding LGE Image in **c2** suggest f ibrofatty changes in this region (from Babu-Narayan et al. [20], with permission)

All these data presented on long-term follow up in patients after repair of ToF indicate an excellent life expectancy, but a significant morbidity. This morbidity increases with the longer time difference between repair and follow-up examination. The main causes for reoperation are problems with the RVOT. As prevention for these problems, the pulmonary valve annulus should be left as intact as possible.

Attention should be not only focused on the right side of the heart but also on the adverse interaction between RV and LV. LV dysfunction is one of the strongest indicators associated with a low functional class and occurrence of arrhythmia.

References

1. Lindinger A, Schwedler G, Hense HW (2010) Prevalence of congenital heart defects in newborns in Germany. Results of the First Registration Year of the PAN Study. Klin Padiatr 222:321-326
2. Bertranou FG, Blackstone EH, Hazelrig JB et al (1978) Life expectancy without surgery in Tetralogy of Fallot. Am J Cardiol 42:458-66
3. Rygg IH, Olesen K, Boesen I (1971) The life history of Tetralogy of Fallot. Dan Med Bull 18(Suppl I):25-30
4. Samánek M (1992) Children with congenital heart disease: probability of natural survival. Pediatr Cardiol 13:152-15
5. Campbell M (1972) Natural history of cyanotic malformations and comparison of all common cardiac malformations. Br Heart J 34:3-8
6. White PD, Sprague H (1929) The Tetralogy of Fallot. Report of a case in a noted musician who lived until his 60th year. JAMA 92:787-791

7. Kirklin JW, Wallace RB, McGoon DC (1965) Early and late results after intracardiac repair of Tetralogy of Fallot: 5-year review of 337 patients. Ann Surg 162:578-589

8. Lindberg HL, Saatvedt K, Seem E et al (2011) Single-center 50 years' experience with surgical management of Tetralogy of Fallot. Eur J Cardiothorac Surg 40:538-542

9. Bacha EA, Scheule AM, Zurakowski D et al (2001) Long-term results after early primary repair of Tetralogy of Fallot. J Thorac Cardiovasc Surg 122:154-161

10. Murphy JG, Gersh BJ, Mair DD et al (1993) Long-term outcome in patients undergoing surgical repair of Tetralogy of Fallot. Engl J Med 329:593-599

11. Nollert G, Fischlein T, Bouterwek S et al (1997) Long-term survival in patients with repair of tetralogy of Fallot: 36-year follow-up of 490 survivors of the first year after surgical repair. J Am Coll Cardiol 5:1374-1383

12. Oechslin EN, Harrison DA, Harris L et al (1999) Reoperation in adults with repair of Tetralogy of Fallot: indications and outcomes. J Thorac Cardiovasc Surg 118:245-251

13. Park CS, Lee JR, Lim HG et al (2010) The long-term result of total repair for Tetralogy of Fallot. Eur J Cardiothorac Surg 38:311-317

14. Gerling C, Rukosujew A, Kehl HG et al (2009) Do the age of patients with Tetralogy of Fallot at the time of surgery and the applied surgical technique influence the reoperation rate? Herz 34:155-160

15. Broberg CS, Aboulhosn J, Mongeon FP et al (2011) Alliance for Adult Research in Congenital Cardiology (AARCC). Prevalence of left ventricular systolic dysfunction in adults with repaired Tetralogy of Fallot. Am J Cardiol 107:1215-1220

16. Geva T, Sandweiss BM, Gauvreau K et al (2004) Factors associated with impaired clinical status in long-term survivors of Tetralogy of Fallot repair evaluated by magnetic resonance imaging. J Am Coll Cardiol 43:1068-1074

17. Knauth AL, Gauvreau K, Powell AJ et al (2008) Ventricular size and function assessed by cardiac MRI predict major adverse clinical outcomes late after Tetralogy of Fallot repair. Heart 94:211-216

18. Khairy P, Harris L, Landzberg MJ et al (2008) Implantable cardioverter defibrillators in Tetralogy of Fallot. Circulation 117:363-370

19. Davlouros PA, Kilner PJ, Hornung TS et al (2002) Right ventricular function in adults with repaired Tetralogy of Fallot assessed with cardiovascular magnetic resonance imaging: detrimental role of right ventricular outflow aneurysms or akinesia and adverse right-to-left ventricular interaction. J Am Coll Cardiol 40:2044-2052

20. Babu-Narayan SV, Kilner PJ, Li W et al (2006) Ventricular fibrosis suggested by cardiovascular magnetic resonance in adults with repaired Tetralogy of Fallot and its relationship to adverse markers of clinical outcome. Circulation 113:405-413

Tetralogy of Fallot: the Failing Right Ventricle

7

Folkert J. Meijboom and Barbara Mulder

7.1 Background: Possible Causes of RV Dysfunction in Tetralogy of Fallot

In the most common form of ToF – a combination of a large, unrestrictive ventricular septal defect (VSD), an overriding aorta and a severe right ventricular outflow tract obstruction (RVOTO) – the prenatal loading conditions are similar to that of the normal heart, but from birth the right ventricle (RV) has abnormal loading conditions.

Directly after birth, when the afterload for the RV drops in the normal heart, the afterload for the RV rises because the large, unrestrictive VSD exposes the RV to the same afterload as the left ventricle. This afterload is increased compared to the prenatal situation because the low-resistance placental circulation is no longer part of the systemic circulation. Higher afterload will result in increase of wall thickness – RV hypertrophy – in order to reduce wall stress. Increase in RV hypertrophy in the already narrowed RVOT will lead to a decrease of the lumen in this part of the RV. This will increase right-to-left shunting at the expense of pulmonary blood flow. In various degrees of RVOTO the afterload to LV and RV are identical.

On top of possible damage from the pressure overload, RV myocardium may be damaged further by hypoxemia, due to the fact that the blood that enters the coronary arteries is substantially desaturated. The pressure overload persists until surgical correction is performed. Surgery invariably consists of closure of the VSD and – depending on the exact anatomy of the RVOT, size of pulmonary annulus, morphology and function of the pulmonary valve and

F.J. Meijboom (✉)
Departments of Cardiology and Pediatric Cardiology, University Medical Center Utrecht,
Utrecht, The Netherlands
e-mail: f.j.meijboom@umcutrecht.nl

M. Chessa, A. Giamberti (eds.), *The Right Ventricle in Adults with Tetralogy of Fallot,*
© Springer-Verlag Italia 2012

size of main pulmonary artery and its branches – desobstruction of the RVOT.

The age at which surgical correction is performed has changed considerably over the past decades, throughout the history of intracardiac surgery, which now covers almost 60 years [1]. In the early years, surgery in neonates or infants was not possible because of technical reasons and very high risks. Childhood mortality for ToF was very high in this period. Patients who survived either had a very favorable anatomy and could survive without surgery, or received an arterial-to-pulmonary shunt first. These shunts were often named after the people who first performed or described them, like the Blalock-Taussig shunt from left subclavian artery to left pulmonary artery, the Pott's anastomosis from the descending aorta to left pulmonary artery and the Waterston anastomosis, from the ascending aorta to right pulmonary artery. By these shunts, pulmonary blood flow was guaranteed and surgical correction could be postponed for many years. This meant that the exposure of the RV to pressure overload, with ongoing damage to the myocardium, was present during all these years.

At the time of corrective surgery, the RV myocardium is, as a rule, severely hypertrophied. Extensive myocardectomy is usually performed, especially in the RVOT, in order to desobstruct it. Quite often, the amount of relief of the RVOTO achieved by myectomy alone is not sufficient and an adequate size of RVOT can only be ascertained by cutting open the RVOT from the anterior and inserting an enlargement patch. This means that part of the functioning myocardium is replaced by non-contractile tissue. The remaining part of the RV myocardium, damaged by the long-standing pressure overload and coronary blood flow with less oxygenated blood in the years before surgery, and by the direct scarring due to extensive myocardectomy, has to cope with the postoperative loading conditions.

In native ToF a narrow pulmonary annulus, a stenosed valve and a narrow main pulmonary artery (MPA) are very common. At surgery this has to be tackled too. Widening of the annulus and main pulmonary artery is often achieved by cutting open the pulmonary annulus and MPA from anterior and placing a patch over the annulus and MPA. The most commonly used technique is the insertion of one large patch from the RVOT, over the pulmonary annulus, into the MPA, almost to the level of the pulmonary bifurcation. Such a patch is often referred to as transannular patch. In this situation, the pulmonary valve is, by definition, no longer competent and pulmonary regurgitation is the rule.

Directly after surgical correction, the remaining part of the RV myocardium no longer has the increased work load (and wall stress) of the elevated systolic pressure. In a few months – possibly years – remodelling will take place and the RV myocardium will actively become thinner, but initially, when the RV myocardium is still thick, the diastolic properties of the RV will be impaired. This is due to a combination of reduced compliance of the remaining myocardium and non-compliance of the large patches in the RVOT and interventricular septum. The increase in RV volume that takes place during rapid filling in early-diastole will lead to a rapid increase of the RV diastolic pressure. This early-diastolic increase of RV pressures will reduce the pressure difference between the pulmonary artery and the RV, thus limiting the degree of pulmonary regurgitation. The reduced RV compliance must be met by elevation of central venous pressures (CVP), in order to achieve adequate RV filling for a stroke volume good enough for the filling (preload) of the left ventricle, to maintain adequate systemic circulation. Gradually, when the RV myocardium becomes thinner, RV compliance improves, lowering the filling pressures. The elevated CVP will disappear but pulmonary regurgitation will increase.

In the months and years following surgery, thinning of the RV myocardium leads to improved RV compliance. Increase of RV volume in diastole will no longer lead to a rapid increase in RV diastolic pressures. Pulmonary regurgitation (PR) will no longer be limited by a rapid increase of RV pressures due to decreased compliance and the RV is able to accommodate much more regurgitant blood flow than before: the pulmonary regurgitation increases. Since functioning pulmonary valve leaflets are virtually absent since the operation, this may increase to a free (without any obstruction) regurgitation, which may be up to 60% of the stroke volume of the RV. This means a gradual increase of RV volume and a gradual increase of the RV stroke volume, necessary to meet the demands of the systemic circulation: the net forward flow (stroke volume) of the RV – the total forward flow in systole minus the diastolic backflow due to the PR – should equal the stroke volume of the LV.

In the balanced situation months or years after surgery, with a moderate or severe PR, the RV wall, with a myocardium that is damaged by the pre-operative situation, partly consists of contractile myocardium and partly of pericardium or dacron patch material. This damaged RV has to produce a much larger stroke volume than the LV. The chronic volume overload of the RV as a result of chronic PR is detrimental to RV function in the long run, and also has a negative effect on LV function [2]. Initially, in the first years after cardiac surgery, it is generally well tolerated. In infants and children, pulmonary regurgitation – even if this has developed into severe regurgitation – rarely leads to clinical problems.

7.2   Definition of RV Failure and RV Dysfunction

In an extensive review of RV function [3, 4], RV failure is defined as "a complex clinical syndrome that can result from any structural or functional cardiovascular disorder, that impairs the ability of the RV to fill or to eject blood. The cardinal clinical findings are (1) fluid retention, which may lead to peripheral edema and ascites, (2) decreased systolic reserve or low cardiac output, which may lead to exercise intolerance and fatigue and (3) ventricular or atrial arrhythmias."

RV dysfunction refers to abnormalities of RV filling or contraction without reference to signs or symptoms [5]. In clinical use, ejection fraction more or less equals systolic ventricular function [6]. In an experimental setting, ventricular elastance – in other words, end-systolic pressure-volume relationship – is a better parameter and the most reliable index of contractility, both for the left [7, 8] and right ventricle [9–11]. Despite being not the best index, ejection fraction (EF) is widely used as marker for LV function, since there are many studies in acquired cardiology linking EF with hard outcome parameters, like death or heart failure. There are also some studies showing that RV dysfunction, defined as decreased EF, is an independent risk factor in cases where it is secondary to left heart disease [12–16]. However, similar outcome studies in congenital heart disease, where RV is the primarily affected ventricle, are very rare, or rather nonexistent. Despite not being proved by adequately-powered studies, it is generally assumed that RV with a decreased EF is much more likely to fail in the foreseeable future than RV with a normal EF.

The assessment of RV diastolic dysfunction is a real challenge. In the development of LV failure, diastolic dysfunction is thought to be an early marker of diminished LV function that often precedes systolic dysfunction. This is not the case in the development of RV failure. Both in case of increased afterload – RV outflow tract obstruction or development of pulmonary arterial hypertension (PAH) – or increased preload (more RV filling due to pulmonary regurgitation), systolic function usually declines first. However, RV diastolic dysfunction does exist. There are contrasting data regarding the interpretation of markers of RV dysfunction. Greenberg et al. [17] reported that a reduction in the E:A ratio across the TV in children was associated with RV diastolic dysfunction and correlated well with right ventricular enlargement [18]. In children with diastolic restrictive physiology a decreased exercise capacity was reported [19]. In contrast, Gatzoulis et al. [20] showed that a restrictive RV physiology in adults was associated with less severe PR, less RV dilatation and a superior exercise performance.

Since RV and LV are enclosed in one pericardial sac with poor compliance, altered RV hemodynamics will affect the left side of the heart as well. By means of modern echo techniques (like tissue Doppler of 2D strain) LV systolic function is shown to be diminished [21]. Longstanding altered LV function, preoperative cyanosis, a previous shunt and cross-talk with a poorly functioning RV may eventually lead to overt LV dysfunction and failure. This happens not infrequently in older patients with ToF, especially those who have had severely compromised RV function, often for decades. Once LV function has become poor, prognosis of patients is poor. Assessment of LV function is therefore indicated in all patients with ToF.

7.3 RV Failure and RV Dysfunction in Tetralogy of Fallot

In the early days of cardiac surgery, cardiac imaging was less sophisticated and clinical decision-making regarding pulmonary valve replacement (PVR) was largely depending on clinical signs and symptoms. Often PVR was performed in patients with signs of RV failure [22]. Despite the – in the current

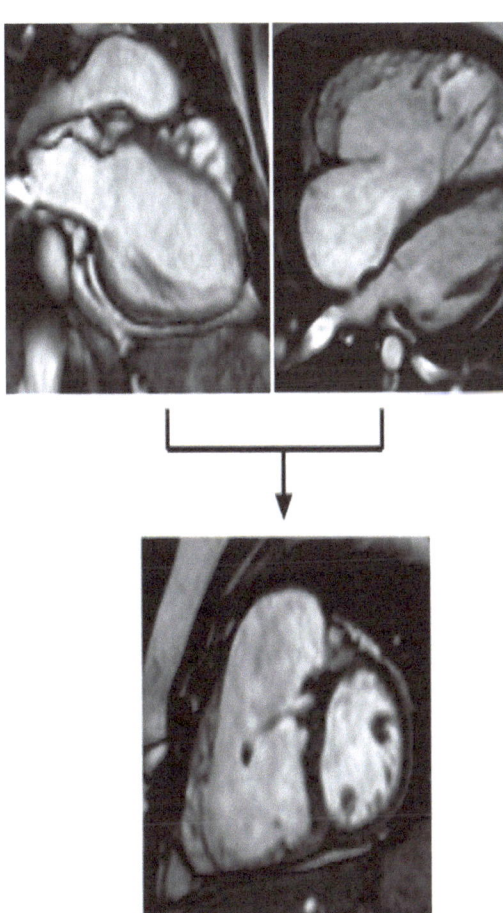

Fig. 7.1 Cine still-frame images of a 2-chamber, a 4-chamber, and a short-axis image. Note the severely dilated right ventricle in the 4-chamber view and the RVOT dilatation in the short-axis image. Multiple short-axis cines from the apex to the base of the heart (or orientated axial) are used to quantify RV and LV function (from Oosterhof et al. [30], with permission)

perspective – crude indications for PVR, the reported long-term outcome is rather good [23, 24]. In many, but not all, patients the clinical signs of RV failure disappeared [25]. It became obvious that PVR had come too late for these patients. This was confirmed by a later study by Therrien et al. [26]: PVR performed in patients with an right ventricular ejection fraction (RVEF) of less than 40% – assessed with radio-nuclide angiography (RNA) – showed no RVEF improvement after PVR. More recently, similar conclusions were drawn from many studies using cardiac magnetic resonance (CMR) for quantification of RV volumes and EF [27, 28], although almost all studies have small sample sizes, without an adequate reference group. Although even the largest RVs decrease in size after PVR, several authors showed that PVR should be performed before certain thresholds of RV volumes are passed, in order to have a chance of normalization of RV volumes: Oosterhof et al. [29] quote an RV EDV index < 160 ml/m2 or RV ESV index < 82 ml/m2 (defining normal volumes as RV EDV index < 108 ml/m2 and RV ESV index < 47 ml/m2) (Fig. 7.1).

Since the risk of irreversible RV dysfunction is substantial and the risk of surgical PVR is low, with a mortality of 1% or less in experienced centers, there is a consensus that postponing PVR until clinical signs of RV failure should be avoided. However, the beneficial effects of early intervention – RV preservation – must be weighed up against the downside: the almost unavoidable degradation of the allograft. This will lead to (numerous) interventions [31, 32]. The detection of RV dysfunction, before clinical signs of failure develop, and defining criteria and cut-off values when to intervene has become a real challenge. So far, the issue of the optimal timing for PVR in a patient with severe PR after ToF repair is not yet entirely settled [33]. This will be extensively discussed in chapter 10.

7.4 Work-up of a Patient with Tetralogy of Fallot with Severe PR in Clinical Practice

The annual outpatient clinic visit contains the following regular components: history, physical examination, electrocardiogram (ECG) and echocardiography. Periodically a formal exercise testing can be done and a CMR is usually performed (in most centers) every 3–5 years and even more on indication [34, 35]. The role of biomarkers in RV dysfunction and RV failure has been looked at in quite a few studies, but so far they do no not play a role in clinical practice [36–39]

7.4.1 History

The history is not very sensitive. The decrease of exercise capacity is so slow and gradual that people may hardly notice and adjust automatically to these slightly altered physical limitations. Often, the first signs of RV failure start to become manifest in adolescence or young adulthood, in a time that many other changes take place in life: end of high school, the first job or starting further education, leaving the parental house, less organized sporting activities and maybe starting a new relationship or marriage. In this turmoil of events it is very hard to point at the RV as the responsible factor for more fatigue or decreased physical condition and very few patients will present with this as a new complaint during their visit. On the other hand, complaints about a decrease in exercise capacity should be taken seriously.

7.4.2 Physical Examination

Physical examination plays a crucial role in the discrimination between RV dysfunction and RV failure. Signs of venous congestion, such as elevated CVP, enlarged liver and peripheral edema may indicate right sided heart failure. Auscultation of the heart provides useful information, especially if changes occur. The normal auscultation of a postoperative ToF is a normal first heart sound, a split second heart sound of which the second part – the pulmonic component P2 – is very soft, if audible at all. There is a low-frequent ejection-type murmur on 2R, stopping before the second heart sound (A2) and a diastolic pulmonary regurgitant murmur. These murmurs may change in time as a result of increasing gradient, increase of the regurgitation or change in compliance of the RV. When the gradient over the RVOT increases, the duration of the ejection murmur increases. If the diastolic decrescendo murmur (representing the pulmonary regurgitation) gets shorter at follow-up, either the regurgitation has increased or RV compliance has decreased (or both). If, apart from the typical PS/PR murmurs, a systolic regurgitation type murmur is heard at 4L, tricuspid regurgitation (TR) should be suspected. A dilating RV – as a result of diminishing RV function – results in progressive TR. In case of normal systolic pressure in the RV, a TR, even when it is severe, is often not heard. If the systolic RV pressure is mildly elevated, a TR murmur can be heard as a holosystolic, mid- to high-frequent regurgitant type murmur on 4L. If this is heard for the first time, extensive assessment of the TV function, including CMR, is advisable.

7.4.3 ECG

Most operated patients have a right bundle branch block (RBBB) with a QRS duration of > 120 msecs after surgery. This is most often a distal RBBB, caused by the RV ventriculotomy and scar in the RVOT. The depolarization of the RVOT is delayed. If the RV dilates, it is often the RVOT that dilates most. Consequently it will take longer to depolarize this enlarged RVOT; the QRS duration will increase. Increase of the QRS duration is a sign of increase in RV size, or decreased function [40]. Rapid progression of the QRS duration or increase to a duration of > 180 msec is an alarm sign, since this is associated with sudden death and ventricular arrhythmias [41-44]. After PVR a beneficial effect on QRS duration has been demonstrated [45, 46], which might be transient.

7.4.4 Chest X-ray

RV size can be seen readily on a chest X-ray. Increase of the cardio-thoracic ratio (CT-ratio) at serial follow-up of anterior-posterior chest X-ray indicates cardiac enlargement; when combined with a lateral chest X-ray RV dilatation can be differentiated reliably from LV dilatation. Although not in the ESC guidelines because of its low sensitivity and specificity, it might be useful to have at least one chest X-ray at an adult age, which can be used for comparison with a new X-ray done at the time that RV dilatation is suspected.

7.4.5   Echocardiography

Echocardiography should be performed regularly during routine follow-up
[47]. Severity of pulmonary regurgitation will be estimated on the basis of
color Doppler and size and function of the RV can be measured. Despite all
efforts and updates of guidelines on how to measure RV function, the reliability of the 2D echo measurements – compared with CMR, which is considered
the best technique – is poor [48]. Dimensions can be measured and compared
with previous measurements if the (recommended) standard cross sections are
used, but transferring these data into RV volumes and EF leads to unreliable
outcomes. The same is true for another often used measurement of RV function: tricuspid annulus planar systolic excursion (TAPSE). There is a poor correlation of TAPSE with absolute values of EF when used in ToF (or other types
of congenital heart disease). Since the measurement is quite straightforward,
standardized and therefore reproducible, it is useful – as is measurement of RV
dimensions with 2D echo – in longitudinal follow-up. Worsening of TAPSE
probably indicates worsening of RV systolic function. RV dilatation is often
associated with development of TR: if TR develops or progresses – to be
assessed with color and continuous wave (CW) Doppler – this should be seen
as an alarm sign, probably indicating worsening of RV function. The CW pattern of TR is helpful in assessment of RV function in longitudinal follow-up
[49]. The relative duration of systole, measured as duration of the TR divided
by the RR interval, is also a useful marker: increase of the relative duration of
systole means decrease of RV function [50]. Newer echo techniques like tissue
Doppler of the RV basal segments, 2D deformation imaging (strain, strain rate)
[21] and 3D echo [51–53] are very promising, but are not established in clinical practice yet.

Diastolic function is judged on the basis of TV inflow patterns with pulsed
Doppler. Interpretation of E and A waves are similar to that of the inflow pattern of the LV and similar normal values are used but clinical significance
remains unclear because long-term outcome studies correlating these findings
with hard end-points are missing. A reliable sign of restrictive physiology is
opening of the PV and antegrade flow in the main PA during atrial contraction,
present at inspiration and at expiration. As stated before there is conflicting
evidence whether restrictive RV physiology is beneficial in the long run or not.

When deterioration of RV systolic function is suspected on the basis of
echocardiography, RV assessment by magnetic resonance imaging (MRI)
should be performed.

7.5   Other Imaging Modalities

RNA, used as the standard for LVEF for a long time, has always been quite
problematic for assessment of RVEF. Comparison of RNA with CMR shows a
very poor correlation [54] and since CMR has been demonstrated to be quite

reliable and robust for assessment of RV volumes and function, RNA is rarely used anymore in clinical practice. Both computed tomography (CT) and CMR can provide very accurate images of RV with reliable quantitative measurements of end-diastolic and end-systolic volumes and consequently reliable calculation of ejection fraction. Since CMR does not use radiation and CMR can quantify blood flow as well – which CT cannot – CMR has become the advanced imaging modality of choice [55]. Echo has its role in the daily routine, being more accessible than CMR in most hospitals, cheaper and less inconvenient for the patient, but clinical decision making will depend largely on CMR imaging.

Invasive assessment of RV function is feasible and accurate, but is not suitable for longitudinal follow-up because of its invasive nature (with risks and discomfort for the patient) and there are no clearly defined cut-off values – based on these invasive measurements – that would help us in the clinical decison making regarding the optimal timing of PVR.

7.5.1 CMR

RV volumes can be measured accurately and quantitatively with CMR [56]. The time resolution of CMR is good enough to establish the maximum volume in end-diastole and the minimal volume at end-systole. From these volumes, EF can be calculated and despite its shortcomings and theoretical considerations that EF is not the best index for RV systolic function, both RV volumes and EF are currently cornerstones in the clinical decision making regarding PVR. Many discussions in the past years focussed on cut-off points: when – at which RV volume corrected for body surface area (BSA) – should one propose PVR? This issue will be discussed extensively in chapter 10, dedicated to PVR [57].

RV volumes should not only be indexed for BSA – which is clinical practice nowadays – but also for sex and race. The latter is not yet routinely done, but Kawut et al. [58] showed substantial differences in normal values of RV volumes between races and sexes. It is not only the absolute and indexed value of the RV volume that is important in clinical decision making, it is also the shape of the RV [59]. During corrective surgery, RVOT is often enlarged with a (transannular) patch. This patch is usually made of pericardium, which has the tendency to dilate over time. These patches can become so dilated that a large part of the RV consists of an aneurysm of the RVOT; a large non-contractile sac on top of the remaining contracting part of the RV (Fig. 7.2).

This large aneurysm contributes to the volume of RV, but not to the contractile function. If function is expressed as EF, calculated from end-diastolic and end-systolic volumes, a poor EF can be measured even if the contractile part of the RV, the remaining RV myocardium, performs normally. Consequently, EF should be used with caution in clinical decision-making regarding PVR.

The shape of the RVOT aneurysm, best assessed with CMR, is important

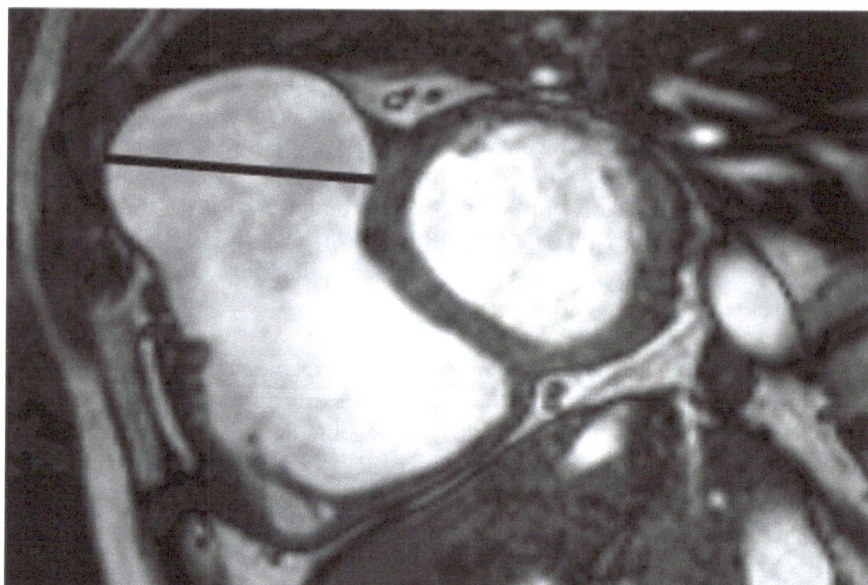

Fig. 7.2 Steady-state free precession cine image obtained in a patient who underwent correction for ToF demonstrates sagittal axis of RVOT. End-diastolic frame depicts RVOT aneurysm. Diameter (*line*) of RVOT measures 5.2 cm (from Oosterhof et al. [60], with permission)

for another reason: the shape of the RVOT prior to PVR correlated with the degree of PR 1 year postoperatively [29]. The more distorted the RVOT, the more severe PR after 1 year. More severe PR after 1 year is strongly associated with decreased longevity of the inserted valve and a shorter duration until yet another PVR is indicated. The angle between RVOT and MPA is also associated with the severity of PR one year after PVR. Therefore, CMR is important not only for quantitative RV volumes, but also for exact shape of the RVOT and geometry of the connection between RV and MPA. The latter requires more elaborate imaging processing, but worth the effort: 3D casts of the RVOT and MPA have proven to be very valuable [61, 62]. Since dilatation and distortion of the RVOT is a gradual process that takes place over time, serial CMR will be valuable. Apart from discussion of what the cut-off value should be in terms of RV volumes for PVR in these patients, above-cited studies provide other reasons not to postpone PVR until the RVOT is substantially dilated and distorted. Viability of the RV myocardium can be assessed with CMR delayed enhancement techniques. Regional differences are often found, but clinical and prognostic significance of these findings is currently largely unknown (Fig. 7.3).

Scarring has been observed in the right ventricle of patients after correction for ToF, most likely as a result of initial repair [60]. These surgery-related scars may contribute to the development of ventricular tachycardias.

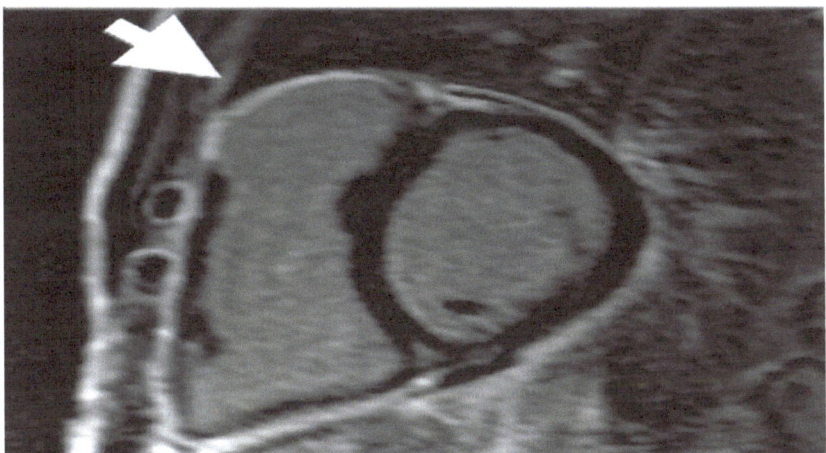

Fig. 7.3 This figure shows delayed enhancement images of the right ventricle (*arrow*). Right ventricular scarring can be observed beginning in the RVOT probably as a result of RV or transannular patching during initial repair. Delayed enhancement is also observed in the posterior alignment of the right ventricle to the left ventricle (from Oosterhof et al. [30], with permission)

Evaluation of cardiac function during stress (physical or pharmacological) allows us to detect ventricular dysfunction, which may not be present at rest (decreased cardiac reserve [63]). However, clinical implementation of the provided parameters needs to be evaluated.

7.6   Conclusion

Assessment of right ventricular function is as difficult as it is crucial in the follow-up of patients with ToF. Understanding of RV physiology, and its adaptation to altered loading conditions, is important. RV failure is a clinical condition that is easy to recognize, but we aim at seeing as few patients as possible in this condition in our follow-up. Imaging – echocardiography and even more important CMR – is necessary to discriminate between adequate adaptation of the RV to altered loading, most often moderate to severe PR, and RV dysfunction. Various aspects of RV dysfunction should be understood and taken into account when PVR is considered. The discussion about when to intervene is not yet concluded. There is also no consensus in terms of aims of an intervention, i.e. PVR: should normality of the RV be aimed for and are multiple interventions in a lifetime – all with a certain inherent risk – justified to achieve this normality, or should other aims be set? So far we do not have the data to conclude this ongoing discussion and years – if not decades – of data-gathering and research on RV function will be necessary before solid, evidence-based advice on optimal timing of interventions can be given.

References

1. Lillehei CW, Cohen M, Warden HE et al (1955) Direct vision intracardiac surgical correction of the tetralogy of Fallot, pentalogy of Fallot, and pulmonary atresia defects; report of first ten cases. Ann Surg 142:418-445
2. Davlouros PA, Kilner PJ, Hornung TS et al (2002) Right ventricular function in adults with repaired tetralogy of Fallot assessed with cardiovascular magnetic resonance imaging: detrimental role of right ventricular outflow aneurysms or akinesia and adverse right-to-left ventricular interaction. J Am Coll Cardiol 40:2044-2052
3. Haddad F, Hunt SA, Rosenthal DN, Murphy DJ (2008) Right ventricular function in cardiovascular disease, part I: Anatomy, physiology, aging, and functional assessment of the right ventricle. Circulation 117:1436-48
4. Haddad F, Doyle R, Murphy D, Hunt SA (2008) Right ventricular function in cardiovascular disease, Part II: Pathophysiology, clinical importance, and management of right ventricular failure. Circulation 117:1717-1731
5. Sheehan F, Redington A (2008) The right ventricle: anatomy, physiology and clinical imaging. Heart 94:1510-1515
6. Voelkel NF, Quaife RA, Leinwand LA et al (2006) Right ventricular function and failure: Report of a national heart, lung, and blood institute working group on cellular and molecular mechanisms of right heart failure. Circulation 114:1883-1891
7. Suga H, Sagawa K, Shoukas AA (1973) Load independence of the instantaneous pressure-volume ratio of the canine left ventricle and effects of epinephrine and heart rate on the ratio. Circ Res 32:314-322
8. Starling MR, Walsh RA, Dell'Italia LJ et al (1987) The relationship of various measures of end-systole to left ventricular maximum time-varying elastance in man. Circulation 76:32–43
9. Redington AN, Gray HH, Hodson ME et al (1988) Characterisation of the normal right ventricular pressure-volume relation by biplane angiography and simultaneous micromanometer pressure measurements. Br Heart J 59:23-30
10. Brown KA, Ditchey RV (1988) Human right ventricular end-systolic pressure-volume relation defined by maximal elastance. Circulation 78:81-91
11. Dell'Italia LJ, Walsh RA (1988) Application of a time varying elastance model to right ventricular performance in man. Cardiovasc Res 22:864-874
12. de Groote P, Millaire A, Foucher-Hossein C et al (1998) Right ventricular ejection fraction is an independent predictor of survival in patients with moderate heart failure. J Am Coll Cardiol 32:948-954
13. Polak JF, Holman BL, Wynne J et al (1983) Right ventricular ejection fraction: an indicator of increased mortality in patients with congestive heart failure associated with coronary artery disease. J Am Coll Cardiol 2:217-224
14. Ghio S, Gavazzi A, Campana C et al (2001) Independent and additive prognostic value of right ventricular systolic function and pulmonary artery pressure in patients with chronic heart failure. J Am Coll Cardiol 37:183-188
15. Mendes LA, Dec GW, Picard MH et al (1994) Right ventricular dysfunction: an independent predictor of adverse outcome in patients with myocarditis. Am Heart J 128:301-307
16. Haddad F, Fisher P, Pham M et al (2009) Right ventricular dysfunction predicts poor outcome following hemodynamically compromising rejection. J Heart Lung Transplant 28:312-319
17. Greenberg SB, Shah CC, Bhutta ST (2008) Tricuspid valve magnetic resonance imaging phase contrast velocity-encoded flow quantification for follow up of tetralogy of Fallot. Int J Cardiovasc Imaging 24(8):861-865
18. Mulder BJ, Vliegen HW, van der Wall EE (2008) Diastolic dysfunction: a new additional criterion for optimal timing of pulmonary valve replacement in adult patient with tetralogy of Fallot? Int J Cardiovasc Imaging 24:867-870
19. Helbing WA, Niezen RA, LeCessie S et al (1996) Right ventricular diastolic function in children with pulmonary regurgitation after repair of tetralogy of Fallot: Volumetric evaluation by Magnetic Resonance mapping. J Am Coll Cardiol 28:1827-1835

20. Gatzoulis MA, Clark AL. Cullen S et al (1995) Right ventricular diastolic function 15 to 35 years after repair of tetralogy of Fallot: Restrictive physiology predicts superior exercise performance. Circulation 91:1775-1781

21. Kempny A, Diller GP, Orwat S et al (2010) Right ventricular-left ventricular interaction in adults with Tetralogy of Fallot: A combined cardiac magnetic resonance and echocardiographic speckle tracking study. Int J Cardiol [Epub ahead of print]

22. Ilbawi MN, Idriss FS, DeLeon SY et al (1986) Long-term results of porcine valve insertion for pulmonary regurgitation following repair of tetralogy of Fallot. Ann Thorac Surg 41:478-82

23. Murphy JG, Gersh BJ, Mair DD et al (1993) Long-term outcome in patients undergoing surgical repair of tertalogy of Fallot. N Engl J Med 329:593-599

24. Nollert G, Fischlein T, Bouterwek S et al (1997) Long-term survival in patients with repair of tetralogy of Fallot: 36 year follow-up of 490 survivors of the first year after surgical repair. J Am Coll Cardiol 30:1374-1383

25. Meijboom FJ, Szatmari A, Deckers JW et al (1995) Cardiac status and health related quality of life long-term after surgical repair of tetralogy of Fallot in infancy and childhood. J Thorac Cardiovasc Surg 110:883-891

26. Therrien J, Siu S, Liu P et al (2000) Pulmonary valve replacement in adults late after repair of tetralogy of Fallot: Are we operating too late? J Am Coll Cardiol 36:1670-1675

27. Frigiola A, Tsang V, Bull C et al (2004) Biventricular response after pulmonary valve replacement for right ventricular outflow tract dysfunction: is age a predictor of outcome? Circulation 118(Suppl 14):S182-190

28. Davlouros PA, Karatza AA, Gatzoulis MA, Shore DF (2004) Timing and type of surgery for severe pulmonary regurgitation after repair of tetralogy of Fallot. Int J Cardiol 97(Suppl 1):91-101

29. Oosterhof T, van Straten A, Vliegen HW et al (2007) Preoperative thresholds for pulmonary valve replacement in patients with corrected tetralogy of Fallot using cardiovascular magnetic resonance. Circulation 116:545-551

30. Oosterhof T, Mulder BJM, Vliegen HW, de Roos A (2006) Cardiovascular magnetic resonance in the follow-up of patients with corrected tetralogy of Fallot: A review. Am Heart J 151:265–272

31. Oosterhof T, Meijboom FJ, Vliegen HW et al (2006) Long-term follow-up of homograft function after pulmonary valve replacement in patients with tetralogy of Fallot. European Heart J 27:1478-1484

32. Oosterhof T, Hazekamp MG, Mulder BJ (2009) Opportunities in pulmonary valve replacement. Expert Rev Cardiovasc Ther 7:1117-1122

33. van der Wall EE, Mulder BJ (2005) Pulmonary valve replacement in patients with tetralogy of Fallot and pulmonary regurgitation: early surgery similar to optimal timing of surgery? Eur Heart J 26:2614-2615

34. Baumgartner H, Bonhoeffer P, De Groot NM et al, Task Force on the Management of Grown-up Congenital Heart Disease of the European Society of Cardiology (ESC) (2010) ESC Guidelines for the management of grown-up congenital heart disease (new version 2010). Eur Heart J 31:2915-2957

35. Silversides CK, Marelli A, Beauchesne L et al (2010) Canadian Cardiovascular Society 2009 Consensus Conference on the management of adults with congenital heart disease: executive summary. Can J Cardiol 26:143-150

36. Book WM, Ilott BJ, McConnell M (2005) B-type natriuretic peptide levels in adults with congenital heart disease and right ventricular failure. Am J Cardiol 95:545-546

37. Oosterhof T, Tulevski I, Vliegen HW et al (2006) Effects of volume and/or pressure overload secondary to congenital heart disease (Tetralogy of Fallot or pulmonary stenosis) on right ventricular function using cardiovascular magnetic resonance and B-type natriuretic peptide levels. Am J Cardiol 97:1051-1055

38. Tulevski II, Groenink M, Van der Wall EE et al (2001) Increased brain and atrial natriuretic peptides in patients with chronic right ventricular pressure overload (correlation between plasma neurohormones and right ventricular dysfunction). Heart 86:27-30

39. Bolger AP, Sharma R, Li W et al (2002) Neurohormonal activation and the chronic heart failure syndrome in adults with congenital heart disease. Circulation 106:92-99
40. Neffke JG, Tulevski II, van der Wall EE et al (2002) ECG determinants in adult patients with chronic right ventricular pressure overload caused by congenital heart disease: relation with plasma neurohormones and MRI parameters. Heart 88:266-270
41. Gatzoulis MA, Balaji S, Webber SA et al (2000) Risk factors for arrhythmia and sudden death in repaired tetralogy of Fallot: a multi-centre study. Lancet 356:975-981
42. Gatzoulis MA, Till JA, Somerville J, Redington AN (1995) Mechanoelectrical interaction in tetralogy van Fallot. QRS prolongation relates to right ventricular size and predicts malignant ventricular arrhytmias and sudden death. [see comments] Circulation 92:231-237
43. Harrison DA, Harris L, Siu SC et al (1997) Sustained ventricular tachycardia in adult patients late after repair of tetralogy of Fallot. J M Coll Cardio 30:1368-1373
44. El Rahman M, Abul-Khaliq H, Vogel M et al (2000) Relation between right ventricular enlargement, QRS duration, and right ventricular function in patients with tetralogy of Fallot and pulmonary regurgitation after surgical repair. Heart 84:416-420
45. Oosterhof T, Vliegen HW, Meijboom FJ et al (2007) Long-term effect of pulmonary valve replacement on QRS duration in patients with corrected tetralogy of Fallot. Heart 93:506-509
46. Scherptong RW, Hazekamp MG, Mulder BJ et al (2010) Follow-up after pulmonary valve replacement in adults with tetralogy of Fallot: association between QRS duration and outcome. J Am Coll Cardiol 56:1486-1492
47. Lopez L, Cohen MS, Anderson RH et al (2010) Unnatural history of the right ventricle in patients with congenitally malformed hearts. Cardiol Young 20(Suppl 3):107-112
48. Helbing WA, Bosch HG, Maliepaard C et al (1995) Comparison of echocardiographic methods with magnetic resonance imaging for assessment of right ventricular function in children. Am J Cardiol 76:589-594
49. Mertens LL, Friedberg MK (2010) Imaging the right ventricle–current state of the art. Nat Rev Cardiol 7:551-563
50. Friedberg MK, Silverman NH (2007) The systolic to diastolic duration ratio in children with hypoplastic left heart syndrome: a novel Doppler index of right ventricular function. J Am Soc Echocardiogr 20:749-755
51. van der Zwaan HB, Geleijnse ML, Soliman OI et al (2011) Test-retest variability of volumetric right ventricular measurements using real-time three-dimensional echocardiography. J Am Soc Echocardiogr
52. van der Zwaan HB, Helbing WA, Boersma E et al (2010) Usefulness of real-time three-dimensional echocardiography to identify right ventricular dysfunction in patients with congenital heart disease. Am J Cardiol 106:843-508
53. van der Zwaan HB, Helbing WA, McGhie JS et al (2010) Clinical value of real-time three-dimensional echocardiography for right ventricular quantification in congenital heart disease: validation with cardiac magnetic resonance imaging. J Am Soc Echocardiogr 23:134-140
54. Rees S, Somerville J, Warnes C et al (1988) Comparison of magnetic resonance imaging with echocardiography and radionuclide angiography in assessing cardiac function and anatomy following Mustard's operation for transposition of the great arteries. Am J Cardiol 61:1316-1322
55. Kilner PJ, Geva T, Kaemmerer H et al (2010) Recommendations for CMR in adults with congenital heart disease from the respective working groups of the European Society of Cardiology. Eur Heart J 31:794-805
56. Tulevski II, Dodge-Khatami A, Groenink M et al (2003) Right ventricular function in congenital cardiac disease: noninvasive quantitative parameters for clinical follow-up. Cardiol Young 13:397-403
57. Geva T (2011) Repaired tetralogy of Fallot: the roles of cardiovascular magnetic resonance in evaluating pathophysiology and for pulmonary valve replacement decision support. J Cardiovasc Magn Reson 20:13-19
58. Kawut SM, Lima JA, Barr RG et al (2011) Sex and race differences in right ventricular structure and function: the multi-ethnic study of atherosclerosis-right ventricle study. Circulation 123:2542-2551

59. Mulder BJ, van der Wall EE (2009) Tetralogy of Fallot: in good shape? Int J Cardiovasc Imaging 25:271-275
60. Oosterhof T, Mulder BJ, Vliegen HW, de Roos A (2005) Corrected tetralogy of Fallot: delayed enhancement in right ventricular outflow tract. Radiology 237:868-871
61. Nordmeyer J, Tsang V, Gaudin R et al (2009) Quantitative assessment of homograft function 1 year after insertion into the pulmonary position: impact of in situ homograft geometry on valve competence. Eur Heart J 30:2147-2154
62. Grosse-Wortmann L, Redington A (2009) Doing the right thing at the right time: is there more to pulmonary valve replacement than meets the eye? Eur Heart J 30:2076-2078
63. Tulevski II, Hirsch A, Dodge-Khatami A et al (2003) Effect of pulmonary valve regurgitation on right ventricular function in patients with chronic right ventricular pressure overload. Am J Cardiol 2:113-116

Imaging Evaluation

8

Claudio Bussadori

8.1 Introduction

Progress in the fields of diagnostic technique, surgical and interventional treatment, anesthesia, postoperative clinical management and general medical care fields has improved the outcome of patients operated upon for congenital diseases. Many of these adult patients are those operated on for ToF, and these patients frequently need re-intervention, mostly related to surgical remodeling of the right ventricle outflow tract (RVOT) such as residual stenosis or, more frequently, pulmonary regurgitation (PR). This condition particularly affects right ventricular function, which could be also impaired by other concomitant conditions such as peripheral pulmonary stenosis and increased pulmonary vascular resistance which worsen PR or any other associated defect, or acquired pulmonary or cardiac diseases. PR and RVOT changes are direct consequences of complete surgical correction of ToF with infundibulectomy and transannular patching; this may result in RVOT aneurysmal dilation and a large pulmonary annulus. This condition may be tolerated for several years, but, depending on its severity, it results in a progressive right ventricular dilation and dysfunction at certain ages. Long standing chronic right ventricular volume overload also affects the right ventricular inflow tract by tricuspid annulus dilation which results in different degrees of tricuspid regurgitation. This further worsens right ventricle dilatation and dysfunction, affecting also left ventricular filling and function. There are several causes of left ventricular dysfunction such as distortion of the interventricular septum which affects interventricular interaction, aortic dilation with aortic regurgitation, ventricular dissynchronicity and

C. Bussadori (✉)
IRCCS Policlinico San Donato, Pediatric and Adult Congenital Heart Center, San Donato
Milanese (Mi), Italy
e-mail: claudiomaria.bussadori@fastwebnet.it

M. Chessa, A. Giamberti (eds.), *The Right Ventricle in Adults with Tetralogy of Fallot,*   91
© Springer-Verlag Italia 2012

reduced left ventricular diastolic filling [1]. Furthermore, right ventricular dilation causes atrial and ventricular tachyarrhythmias, which are considered an important risk factor for sudden death in this type of patient [2]. Imaging examination in adult postoperative status with PR should address the assessment of several indicators of right ventricular function in order to indicate the most appropriate timing for pulmonary valve replacement (PVR). The answer to this question remains one of the most challenging and controversial points for a clinician. Several authors proposed MRI measurements of right ventricular volumes as a main indicator for PVR: an RV end-diastolic volume greater than 170 ml/m² or a RV end-systolic volume greater than 85 ml/m² have been proposed [3] as a cut off for reoperation to obtain substantial right ventricular normalization after surgery. Other authors considering even correlation between right ventricular volume, cardiac output and exercise test changes after PVR, proposed a relatively more aggressive PVR policy (end diastolic volume less than 150 mL/m², and this resulted in: normalization of right ventricular volumes, improvement in biventricular function, and submaximal exercise capacity [4]. MRI is considered the gold standard for measurement of RV [5] volume, but 2D and more recently 3D echocardiography in the hands of an experienced operator may provide a reliable volume measurement [6, 7] together with much other information that may be obtained in a comprehensive echocardiographic exam [8]. Nevertheless, timing for reoperation frequently remains a dilemma, especially considering the young age of most patients and the relative duration of the biological prosthesis implanted. In the decision of setting a measure of right ventricular volumes obtained by MRI or echocardiography should never be considered as a unique indicator, evaluation of a patient operated for ToF and who is a candidate for PVR should include also electrocardiogram (ECG) and Holter recording, thoracic radiography and, in selected patients, cardiac catheterization.

8.2 Echocardiography

8.2.1 Severity of Pulmonary Regurgitation

To evaluate severity and causes of PR, RVOT should be visualized in an appropriate way; the correct echocardiographic windows for this are the parasternal long and short axes. In some cases in adult patients, and especially after thoracotomy, this may be difficult and a RVOT residual obstruction, transannular patch, a RVOT aneurysm or a conduit degeneration may be better observed with an apical view or a subcostal approach.

Initial evaluation of PR severity can be done using color Doppler. Frequently after the application of a transannular patch a severe pulmonary regurgitation appears as a free floating bidirectional flow across the pulmonary annulus.

In this type of severe PR, dilated pulmonary branches and a bouncing main pulmonary artery are commonly observed.

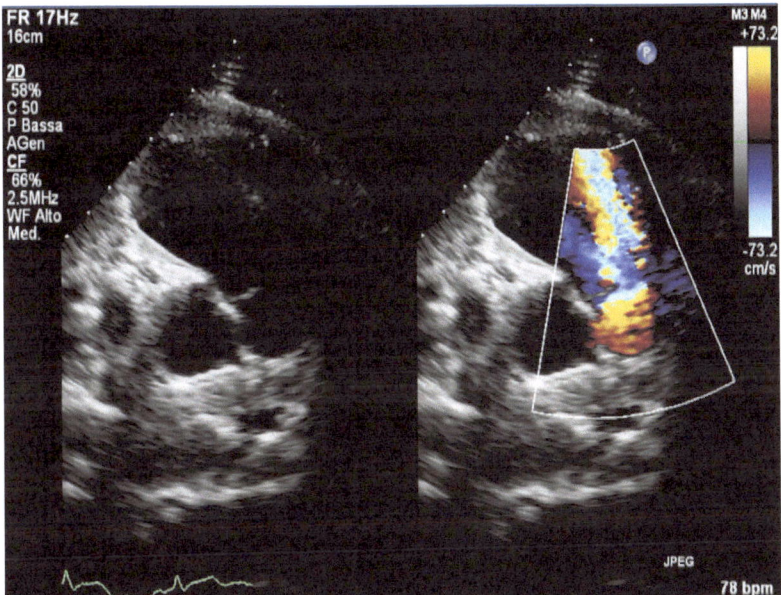

Fig. 8.1 Color flow mapping of a severe pulmonary regurgitation

Several semiquantitative approaches to PR based on color Doppler have been proposed. The simplest one is a mild extension of the reversal flow that sometimes can be observed even in normal patients. On the contrary, a large reversal flow persisting over the mid diastole and invading the RVOT is consistent with a severe PR (Fig. 8.1).

As for other regurgitant flows, extension of a regurgitant color flow map has been used to quantify pulmonary regurgitation. One of the first parameters proposed was obtained indexing the maximum area of the visualized color jet on right parasternal short axis to body surface area. Another index is based on a ratio between the width of the color jet and the annulus area. This last was validated in comparison with angiography [9, 10]. All indexes based on color Doppler have some technical weaknesses and the result could be influenced by the direction of the jet, the gain setting of the color Doppler and the transducer's frequency.

Quantification of PR severity can be assessed more precisely using spectral Doppler. The regurgitant velocity profile expresses the pressure gradient between main pulmonary artery and RV for the whole diastolic time, if pulmonary diastolic pressures are normal, peak velocity is not higher than 1 msec; an indicator of severity is the precocity of the equalization of the two pressures, so in mild PR, the regurgitant flow occupies the whole diastole. Once PR is severe, the reversal flow after an early peak decreases its velocity rapidly (Fig. 8.2). A quantitative assessment of PR severity based on deceleration velocity of the regurgitant flow is pressure half time (PHT): this is the time in

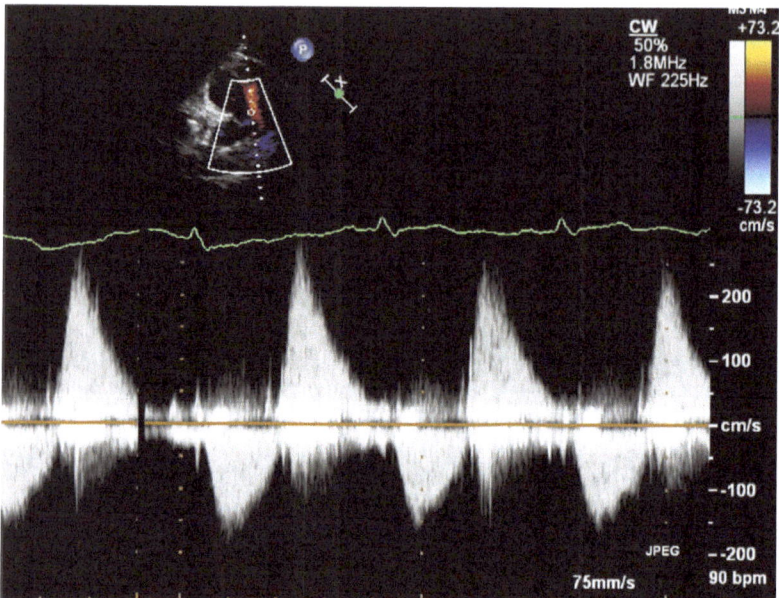

Fig. 8.2 CW Doppler of a severe pulmonary regurgitation, rapid decrease of diastolic reversal flow velocity suggests a rapid increase of diastolic right ventricular pressure

milliseconds taken to reach half of the pressure gradient. This could be easily
measured using continuous wave (CW) Doppler. In a clinical validation study,
PHT was demonstrated to be inversely correlated to the pulmonary regurgitant
fraction measured with MRI [11]. Furthermore, in the same study values of
PHT under 100 msec were a highly specific and significant index of severe PR.
In a recent retrospective study of 135 cases of severe PR, other uncommon
echocardiographic findings were described [12]. The authors found premature
closure of the tricuspid valve in 6.6% of patients, holodiastolic flow reversal
in 3.7%, premature opening of the pulmonary valve in 1.5%, PR with laminar
retrograde flow in 1.5% and very low peak velocity of the PR jet in 1.5%. Even
if very rare, these signs can be considered as an additional indicator of PR
severity.

Spectral Doppler of the pulmonary flow may help to identify other causes
of rapid increasing diastolic pressure in the right ventricle. Other than by
severe PR, this pressure increase could be caused by the myocardial stiffness
frequently observed in the severely hypertrophied and fibrotic right ventricle
of a ToF patient. Because of this restrictive diastolic dysfunction, the regurgitant flow has an early peak and an early finish as in severe PR, but in a restrictive right ventricle the regurgitant flow is attenuated by an increase in diastolic
pressure in mid-late diastole that overrides PA pressure: this gradient is
expressed by an anterograde late diastolic flow through the pulmonary valve
just after atrial contraction (Fig. 8.3). Restrictive physiology, limiting PR, has

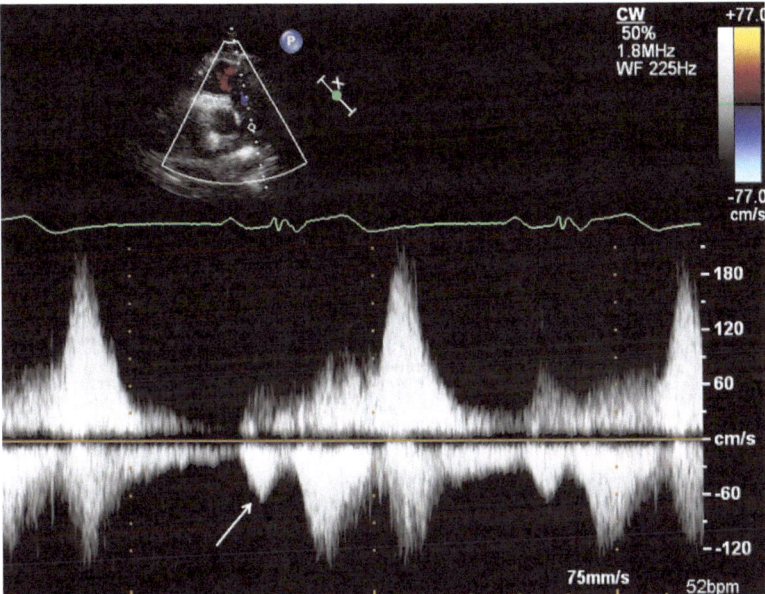

Fig. 8.3 CW Doppler pattern in a restrictive right ventricle with pulmonary regurgitation. The early diastolic retrograde flow suggests a severe PR. The *arrow* indicates the pathognomonic late diastolic anterograde flow after atrial contraction

a protective effect on RV, limiting the effect of volume overload that dilates the right ventricle [13]. Severity of preoperative pulmonic stenosis and older age at time of intervention are the most important predisposing factors to restrictive physiology of the right ventricle [14]. Patients with a restrictive right ventricle have a better performance at exercise test compared to other patients operated on for ToF who have severe PR and do not have this diastolic dysfunction [15]. These restrictive right ventricles have smaller cavity volumes, their chronic concentric hypertrophy causes a rearrangement of fiber orientation similar to that which happens in a systemic right ventricle, with mid wall horizontal fibers that become more influent on ventricular contraction [16]. This increased radial contraction could be the most important determinant of the improved exercise performance mentioned above.

8.2.2   Evaluation of RVOT Morphology and Residual Obstruction

Obstruction of RVOT observed in adult patients operated on for ToF is more frequently caused by degeneration of the valvulated conduit surgically positioned at the time of complete reparation or later to correct PR. Optimal visualization of the obstruction site is sometimes difficult because of suboptimal windows, due to previous sternotomy and conduit calcification. The most appropriate views to visualize RVOT and the pulmonary conduit as well as

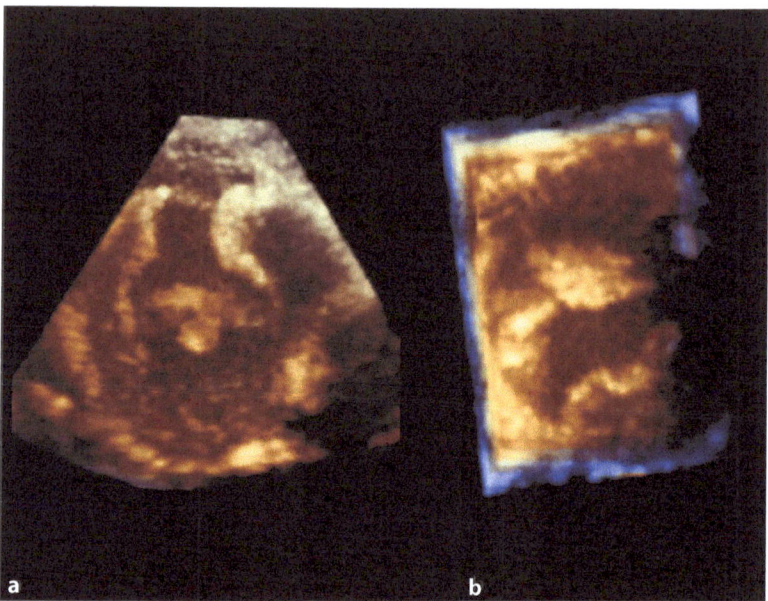

Fig. 8.4 Three dimensional view of a deteriorated prosthetic valve that resulted in a severe pulmonic stenosis. **a** Longitudinal view. **b** Frontal view from the side of the pulmonary artery

analyzing Doppler flow through it, are the parasternal short axis and subcostal view, in both the apical and short axis. The same views could be used to visualize a percutaneously placed valvulated stent. Degenerated prosthetic valves inside the conduit could be visualized appropriately using 3D echocardiography (Fig. 8.4). In patients with percutaneous implanted pulmonary valves it is possible to visualize stent position, prosthetic valve motion (Fig. 8.5) and the flow through them by echocardiography. Difference between type of valvulate can also be easily identified (Fig. 8.6). On the right parasternal short axis, integrity of the interventricular patch should be studied and the eventual residual shunt must be documented (Fig. 8.7). To visualize eventual stent fractures, neither 2D nor 3D is indicated: a fluoroscopy check is the easiest solution (Fig. 8.8). Continuous wave Doppler allows estimation of the pulmonary gradient in order to classify the severity of pulmonic stenosis (Fig 8.9). This measurement may sometimes not be totally reliable for an anomalous anatomy (tunnel stenosis), a suboptimal alignment of the ultrasound beam with pulmonary flow, but above all, in case of pulmonary hypertension (PHT). Increased pressure in the pulmonary artery is not rare in adult ToF patients. In younger patients it can more frequently be due to chronic volume overload caused by palliative shunts or residual intracardiac shunts; in older patients, PHT could be caused by other cardiopulmonary diseases such as pulmonary thromboembolism. PHT leads to an underestimation of the pulmonary stenosis severity and worsens pulmonary regurgitation. Cardiac catheterization is recommended when

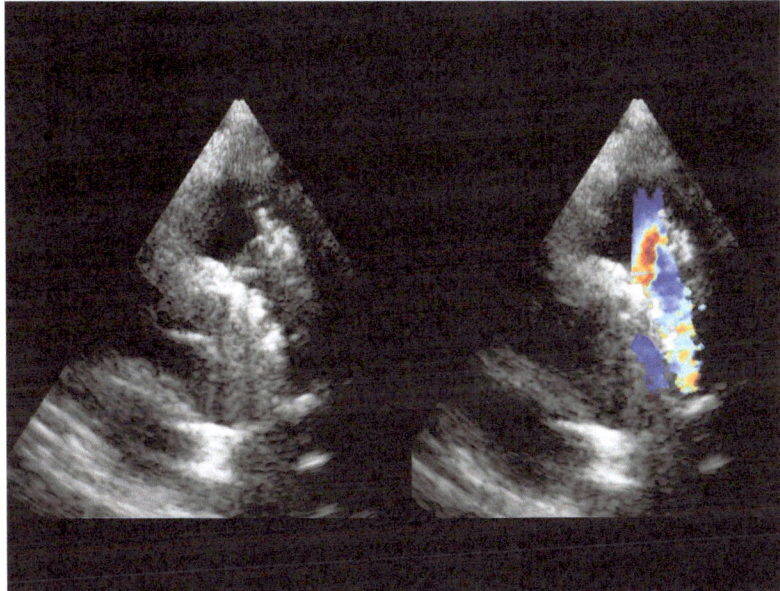

Fig. 8.5 Melody® valve implanted. Prosthetic valve leaflets are visible. At the valvar level Color Flow Mapping shows an acceleration isovelocity area. Anterograde laminar flow through the stent is also visible

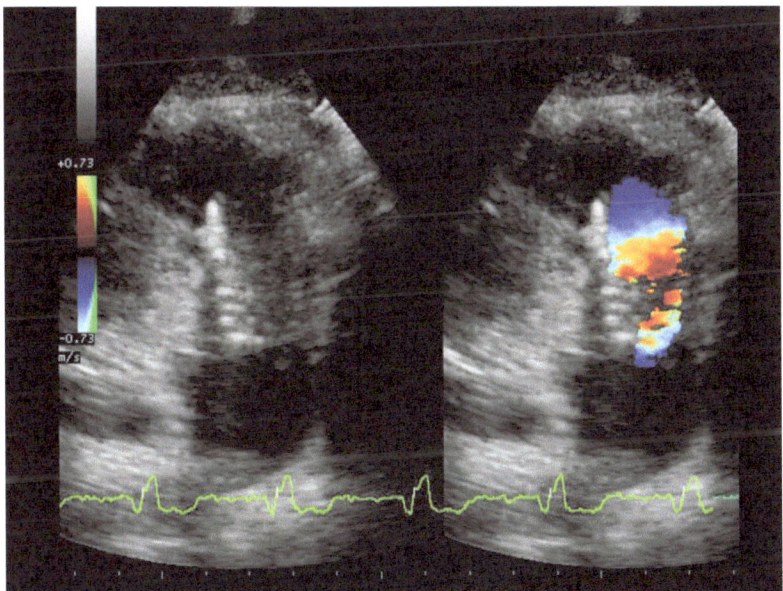

Fig. 8.6 Sapien® valve implanted on RVOT. This prosthesis can be recognized by the shorter and wider shape of the stent

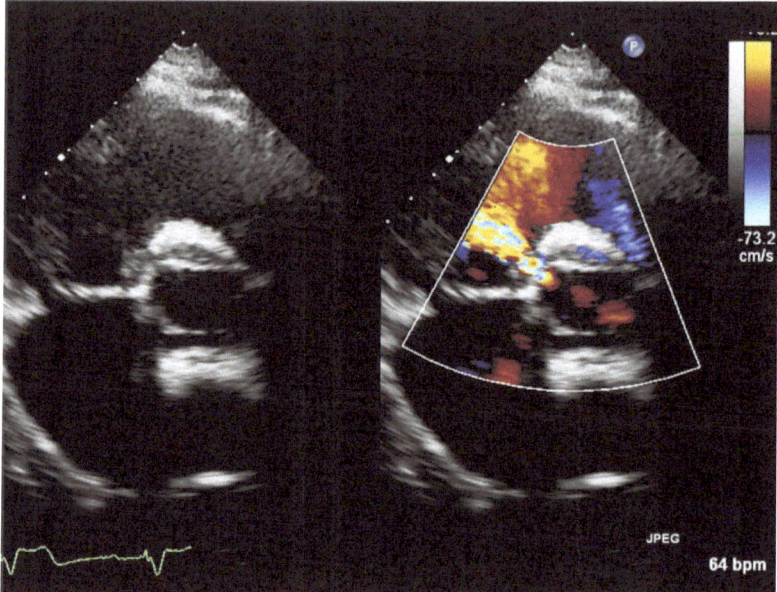

Fig. 8.7 Residual VSD

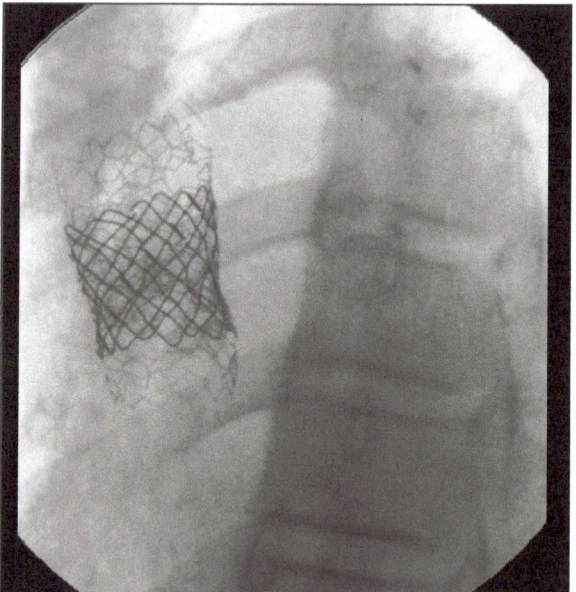

Fig. 8.8 Stent fractures in a Melody® valve

a subestimation of an anterograde gradient due to a difficult alignment is suspected. Indirect confirmation of the severity of the stenosis should be obtained by measuring the peak gradient of tricuspid regurgitation, if visible (Fig. 8.10).

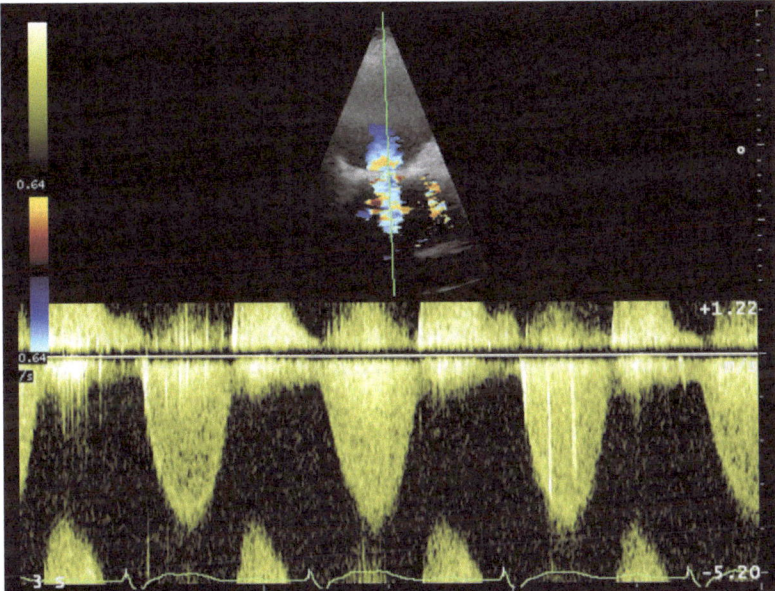

Fig. 8.9 Severe stenosis of a surgically placed pulmonary conduit

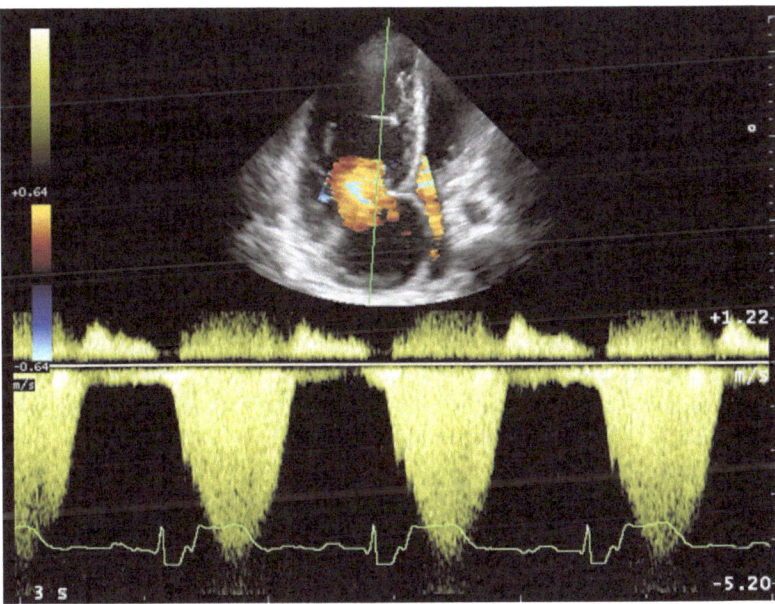

Fig. 8.10 High peak velocity of tricuspid regurgitant flow indicates a severe increase of right ventricular systolic pressure

8.2.3 Right Ventricular Dimension and Function

Before describing in detail all the echocardiographic measurements applied to study the morphology and function of the right ventricle, it is important to consider the peculiarities of the right ventricle of ToF patients and its complex pathophysiological history. Its myocardial structure is congenitally abnormal, hypertrophy and fibrosis are present at birth and generally persist after surgical repair. Consecutively, depending on the surgical option adopted by the surgeon for pulmonic stenosis (conservative or homograft and transannular patch), the right ventricle may conserve or may increase its concentric hypertrophy or start to dilate consequently to severe PR. Most of the patients with RV dysfunction require a surgical implant of a RV to pulmonary artery conduit in order to maintain adequate RV function. A variable period after implantation the conduit may degenerate, mostly causing various degrees of stenosis and consequent pressure overload. At this stage patients should undergo a second surgical intervention to substitute the conduit, or replacement of it with a percutaneous implant of a bovine jugular vein valve mounted on an expandable stent [17]. In all these stages the selection of the appropriate timing for surgery or intervention it is still a debated point. The difficult question for the clinician is when to determine the right moment to indicate valve substitution, not too late when perhaps the right ventricular function has irreversibly deteriorated and its dilatation predisposes to life threatening arrhythmias, but also not too early, considering the young age of the patient and the relative duration of the biological prosthesis. Diagnostic imaging technologies are employed to support the clinician in this scenario; however, determining which is the more appropriate technology or index to evaluate morphology and function of the right ventricle is very difficult, if not impossible. For the complex pathophysiological history mentioned above, with several periods of volume and pressure overload, the shape and function of the ventricle makes it very difficult to reliably estimate the residual ventricular function.

End diastolic volume and end systolic volume of RV are more reliably measured with MRI [3]. This technology overcomes the echocardiographic limitations of poor image quality that are frequent in those patients who have had several surgical interventions. However, due to the complex geometry of the right ventricle, its measurement requires a higher level of expertise compared to left ventricular measurement. In addition, significant intra and inter operator variability for RV volume measurements have been reported [18]. Nowadays MRI evaluation should be recommended for all patients with repaired ToF: nevertheless, this technique cannot provide all the information that can be obtained by a complete echocardiographic exam. Echocardiographic evaluation of the right ventricle should focus on progression of RV dilatation and dysfunction, dilatation of tricuspidal annulus, appearance and worsening tricuspid regurgitation.

Echocardiographic parameters used to evaluate right ventricular function can be divided into geometrical and non geometrical parameters: the former are

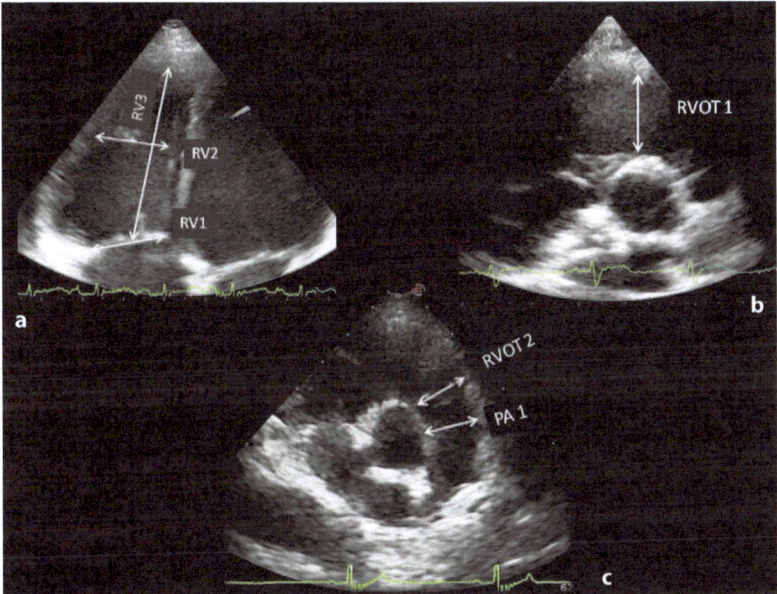

Fig. 8.11 Measurement of the right ventricle as recommended by ASE [19]. **a** Dimension of the right ventricular inflow *RV1* at the tricuspid annulus, *RV2* at the mid ventricular papillary muscle level, *RV3* the longitudinal dimension, all measurements have been executed in diastole. **b** *RVOT1*, right ventricular outflow diameter diastolic and systolic measurements at this level are used to obtain RVOT fractional shortening. **c** *RVOT2*, measurement of pulmonary annulus. *PA1*, pulmonary artery diameter at the sinotubular junction level

based on bidimensional and three-dimensional measurement of RV volumes, the latter, on various technologies including M-mode, myocardial Doppler imaging, tissue Doppler imaging (TDI) and 2D based strain. If bidimensional measures are to be used, one of their major limitations must be considered: most of these echocardiographic dimensional measurements and functional indexes have been created for the purpose of left ventricle examination. However, left ventricular morphology, with its elliptical shape, its modality of contraction and relaxation, with its peculiar twisting and mechanism, is consistently different to that of the right ventricle. Indications for the bidimensional measurement of the right ventricle have been proposed in various guidelines (Fig. 8.11) [19] and original articles [20]. The more commonly used index is fractional area change: this simplified index of systolic function, similar to that performed in left ventricular ejection fraction, is based on the fractional variation of diastolic and systolic area of the right ventricular inflow, measured on an apical four chamber view optimized for the right ventricle (Fig. 8.12). This method is based on a geometric assumption that is insufficient for a ToF operated patient because it does not consider RVOT. The dimension and RVOT function in these patients can be assessed with bidimensional echocardiography

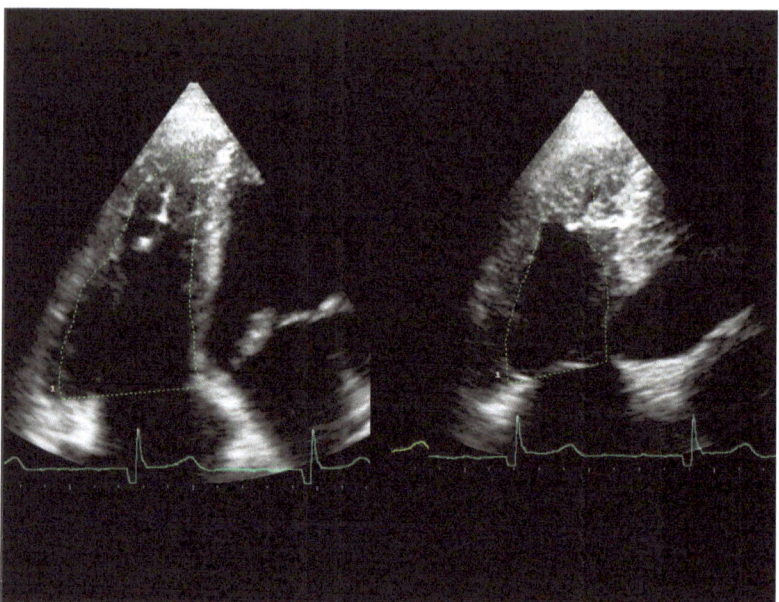

Fig. 8.12 Diastolic and systolic area of the right ventricle traced to measure fractional area change (FAC)

[8]. In this study the radial contraction of the RVOT was assessed by measuring the fractional shortening of the RVOT (FS-RVOT) at the level of the aortic valve (Fig. 8.11b). Furthermore, this confirmed the reliability of two-dimensional echocardiographic study of right ventricular end-diastolic area measured in the apical four-chamber view. When indexed to body surface area this measurement showed good correlation with the same measurement obtained by MR, even following change in time in patients operated upon for ToF.

The right ventricle complex anatomy can be better studied using three dimensional echocardiography (3DE). This technology allows a better assessment of pulmonary valve morphology [21] and characterization of pulmonary flow [22], but underestimations of volumes and ejection fraction (EF) have often been reported [23, 24]. A recent meta analysis of 23 studies including 807 subjects found underestimation of RV volumes and EF by 3DE and identified factors affecting bias. Underestimation was more evident with larger volumes, and in older patients volumes were overestimated and EF was underestimated [25]. 3DE is in continuing technical evolution and operator knowledge and expertise is constantly improving: this will contribute to better understanding, while addressing the elements causing bias in 3DE will help improve its clinical applicability.

Tricuspid annular plane systolic excursion (TAPSE) is very easy and rapid to apply and for this reason is still widely used, but its reliability is controversial [26, 27]. In adults, values of TAPSE lower than 16 mm are suggestive for

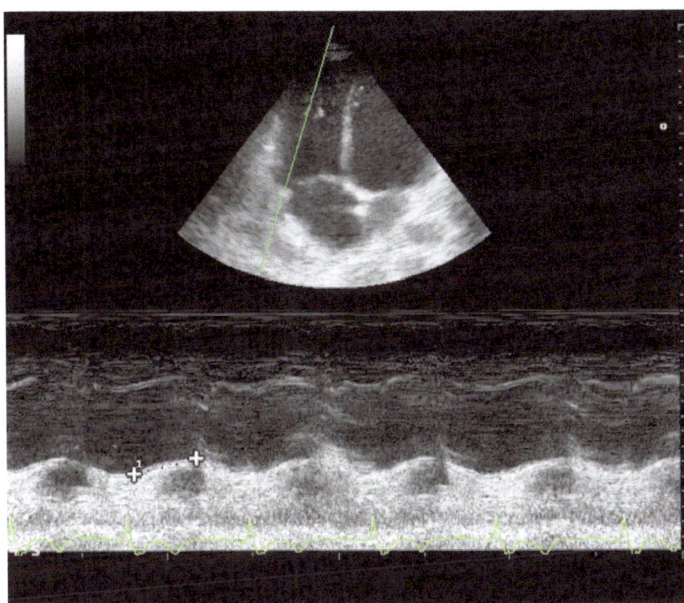

Fig. 8.13 Tricuspid annular plane systolic excursion (TAPSE) measurement, reduced value (10mm) in a patient with right ventricular dysfunction

right ventricular longitudinal dysfunction. In children the absolute value of TAPSE must be indexed to right ventricular longitudinal diameter: values of this ratio lower than 25% suggest longitudinal dysfunction [28, 29]. Unfortunately this index is frequently not reliable in ToF patients, especially when right ventricular hypertrophy is severe. In these patients mid wall circumferential fibers are more hypertrophied and radial contraction becomes the prevalent direction of right ventricular systolic deformation [16] and TAPSE results may underestimate real systolic function.

The Tei Index, known also as the index of myocardial performance (IMP), is a functional index based on Doppler technology that was originally created to study left ventricular global function [30]. Systolic and diastolic times were calculated on the basis of spectral Doppler flow analysis of diastolic and systolic flows (Fig. 8.13). Its application in patients operated on for ToF had some limitations and the literature reports controversial results. In one study of 51 patients after repair of ToF, a strong influence of PR was found, reducing isovolumic relaxation time (IRT) and increasing isovolumic contraction time (ICT) [31]. In addition, reduced RV compliance resulted in decreased IRT and a consequent paradoxically reduced IMP. The authors concluded that this limitation may reduce the sensitivity of the index in recognizing patients with right ventricular dysfunction following corrective surgery of ToF [31]. In a more recent study [18], RV IMP was assessed in 57 adults with repaired ToF and compared with the MRI derived RVEF. These authors found a negative lin-

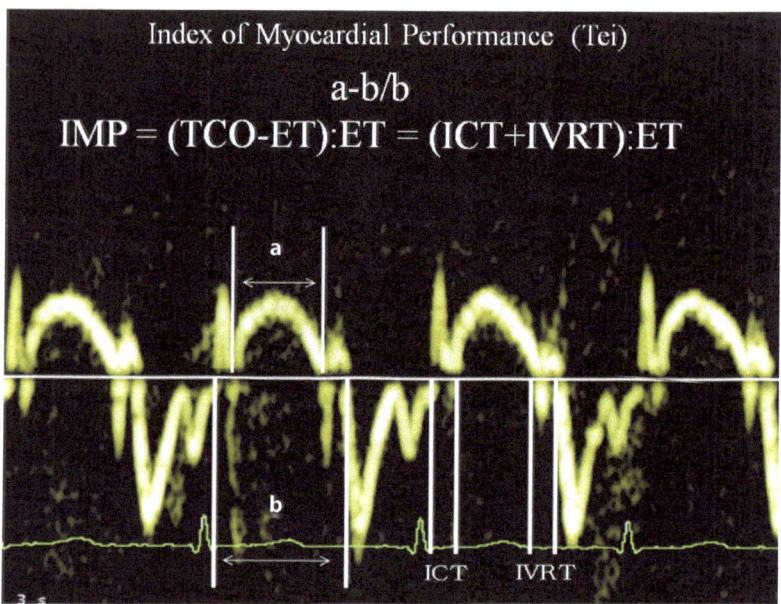

Fig. 8.14 Index of myocardial performance, known as the Tei Index, measured at the tricuspid annulus with TDI. **a** Tricuspid closing to opening time. **b** Ejection time; *ICT,* Isovolumic Contraction Time; *IVRT,* Isovolumic Relaxation Time

ear correlation between the IMP and RVEF (r = 0.73, p <0.001). IMP values of 0.4 were indicative of a EF lower than 35% and, when lower than 0.25, were predictive of RV EF of 50% or higher. Furthermore, using a multivariate regression model these authors demonstrated that IMP was not affected by the degree of pulmonary regurgitation, the presence of tricuspid regurgitation, or QRS duration. In this study right ventricular IMP was calculated deriving interval times with pulsed wave Doppler on tricuspid and pulmonary flow. However, using myocardial Doppler, positioning the sample volume at the tricuspid lateral annulus, data can be derived on consecutive events (Fig 8.14) with the obvious advantage of major precision. A study of 15 children operated on for ToF compared the two methods (PW vs TDI) to measure IMP and demonstrated the superior sensitivity of the TDI based approach [32].

TDI derived data are less load dependent than data derived from Doppler flow analysis. Since this technology is Doppler based, its major limit is angle dependence [33]. Therefore, in the right ventricle, it can be applied only at the tricuspidal annular level or at basal segments. In a group of 124 patients after ToF repair, longitudinal strain TDI based and isovolumic acceleration time (IVA) data obtained at the tricuspid annulus and/or right ventricular basal segments were compared with normal controls (Fig. 8.15) [34]. This study demonstrated the utility of measuring myocardial acceleration during isovolumic contraction, which was lower in all patients compared with controls and correlated with the severity of PR.

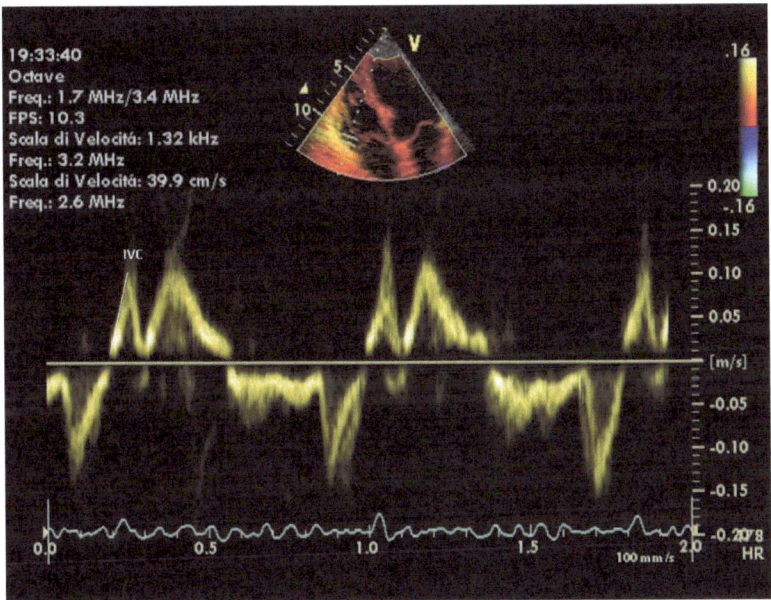

Fig. 8.15 Isovolumic acceleration time at the tricuspid annulus, time is calculated from the beginning of isovolumic contraction curve to its peak

Considering the deformation index, strain and strain rate (SR) are relatively load independent and largely used for direct quantification of systolic and diastolic function. The newest 2D based technology overcomes the limitation of angle dependence and is widely used to study left ventricular function. These are now used in many echolabs to evaluate right ventricular function. 2D strain allows computation of myocardial deformation at any level and in any direction: this is particularly important since in ToF patients right ventricular structures have different patterns of fiber orientation and contraction and the pathophysiology events affect right and left ventricular longitudinal strain, right ventricular transversal strain and left ventricular twist in different ways [35, 36]. Furthermore, with 2D strain it is possible to distinguish longitudinal deformation of the right and left ventricular septum [37, 38].

Use of strain and SR during follow up in these patients allows understanding of changes in pathophysiology and in myocardial structure and function. Children and young adults operated on for ToF, non symptomatic but with various degree of PR, have longitudinal strain of the right lateral wall and right septum, which is lower than normal, and a strong inverse correlation between peak systolic strain of basal lateral wall and QRS duration [35]. This abnormality of right ventricular longitudinal strain is more evident in patients with transannular patches than in those with infundibular patches. Left ventricles in these patients are not only geometrically altered but even deformation parameters, such as longitudinal and radial strain, SR and ventricular

Table 8.1 RV Longitudinal Strain and SR in a young patient with RV dysfunction compared to an age matched control

	Strain (%)				SR (sn.$^{-1}$)		
Segments	RV Dysfunction	Control	P	Segments	RV Dysfunction	Control	P
Basal lateral	−20.7 ± 10.9	−31.8 ± 8.7	0.009	Basal lateral	−1.44 ± 0.9	−1.92 ± 0.52	Ns
Mid lateral	−12.4 ± 7.1	−27.8 ± 5.3	0.0001	Mid lateral	−0.92 ± 0.6	−1.70 ± 0.49	0.001
Apical lateral	−8.6 ± 4.8	−20.3 ± 5.8	0.0001	Apical lateral	−0.55 ± 0.3	−1.05 ± 0.44	0.001
Basal septal	−15.4 ± 8.4	−23.2 ± 4.8	0.001	Basal septal	−1.06 ± 0.56	−1.40 ± 0.6	Ns
Mid septal	−14.0 ± 8.1	−23.3 ± 6.1	0.002	Mid septal	−0.86 ± 0.46	−1.43 ± 0.38	0.022
Apical septal	−12.3 ± 5.3	−25.9 ± 4.7	0.0001	Apical septal	−0.97 ± 0.47	−1.43 ± 0.38	0.04

Ns, not significant.

twist are lower than normal. As all deformation parameters of both ventricles are depressed even at the beginning of the clinical history in these patients, information will be extrapolated following change of these parameters in any patient or even comparing data obtained with that reported in the literature (Table 8.1) [39, 40].

In cases with RV volume overload with a normally structured right ventricle, i.e., atrial septal defect (ASD), there is an increase in right ventricular longitudinal strain and SR that normalizes after closure [38]. On the contrary, in operated ToF, decreasing longitudinal strain of the right ventricular septum (Fig. 8.16) is correlated with RV dilatation and severity of PR. In ToF, RV volume overload occurs in an already altered structure with various degrees of fibrosis; furthermore, longitudinal strain is determined by contraction of longitudinal subendocardial fibers, and these are more damaged during PR because they are very sensitive to wall stress [41]. Low longitudinal strain is found even in restrictive RV ventricles, but in this condition because of the hypertrophy of the transversal fibers mentioned above, a more correct evaluation of systolic function should be done measuring right ventricular transversal strain (Fig. 8.17).

Degeneration of the conduit placed to correct PR in the majority of cases creates a severe stenosis (Fig. 8.18) resulting in an additional systolic wall stress for the right ventricle that may or may not develop further hypertrophy but always results in a further reduction of longitudinal strain and SR.

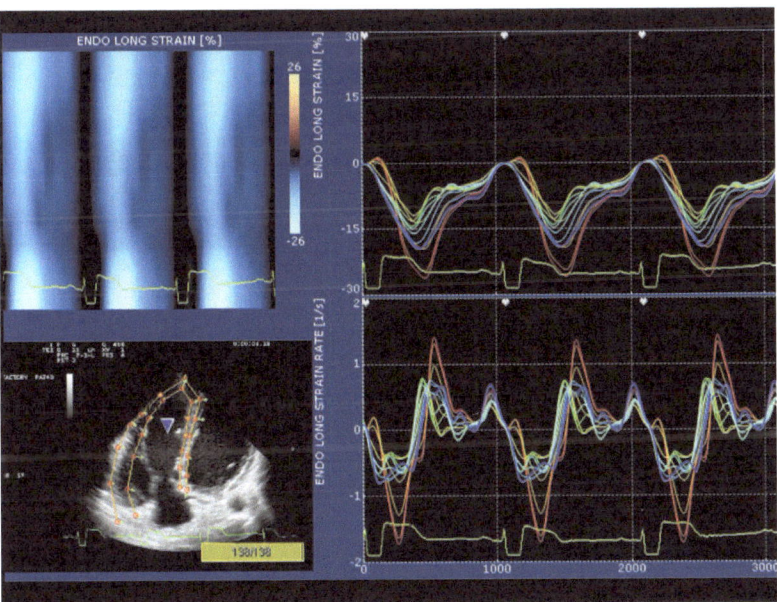

Fig. 8.16 Measurement of right longitudinal strain and SR in a ToF patient 2 years after implant of a Melody valve

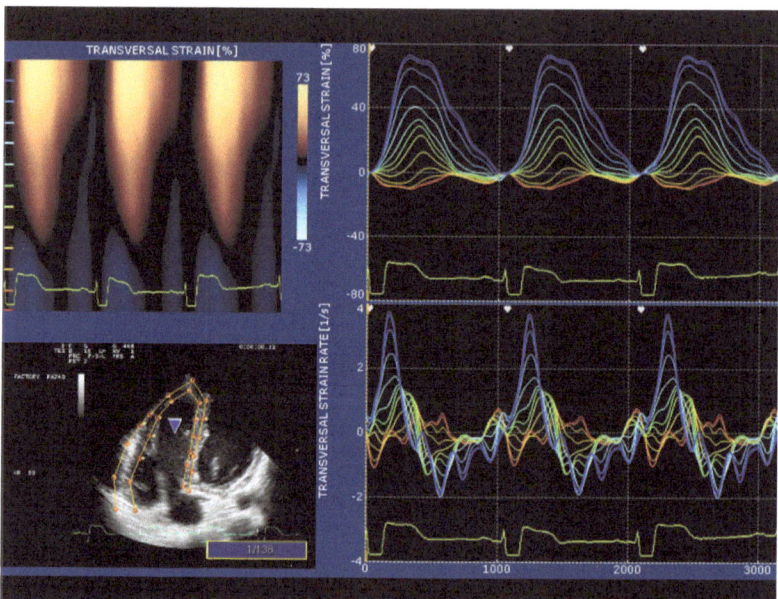

Fig. 8.17 Measurement of right transversal strain and SR in the same patient

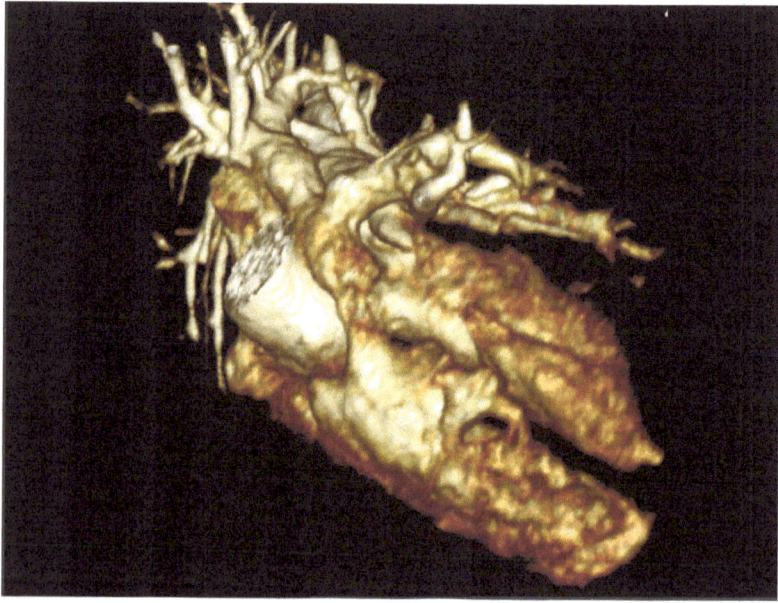

Fig. 8.18 Severe stenosis of a surgically placed pulmonary conduit

In our department most of the patients with stenosis of the conduit are treated with percutaneous implants of biological pulmonary valves mounted on an expandable stent. In these patients, longitudinal strain of the right ventricle increases significantly after percutaneous pulmonary valve (PPV) implant, without reaching values reported by other authors [42, 43]. In our patients, RV longitudinal measurements improve significantly at 24 hours after the procedure and keep improving even between serial controls at 3, 6, and 12 months.

Pre-procedure values of longitudinal strain correlate significantly with the results of the cardio pulmonary exercise test (CPET) and this significant correlation is confirmed at follow up. Particularly, values of longitudinal strain greater than -13% were predictive of a post procedure VO_{2max} greater than 60% of the expected values, with 83% sensitivity and 100% specificity.

Pre-procedure transversal right ventricular strain is directly correlated with RV pressure and gradient, but inversely correlates with the results of CPET even after a successful procedure, at least for short term follow up. This could be explained considering that compensatory radial contraction is more evident in restrictive RV. In this specific pathophysiology, a reduction of gradient could result in improved systolic function at rest, but exercise performance remains impaired because of diastolic dysfunction. In these cases where progressive remodeling of the right ventricle with reduction of hypertrophy occurs, diastolic function may improve together with a patient's performance at CPET in long term follow up.

Nowadays, with the availability of percutaneously implantable pulmonary valves, we need instruments to identify correct timing for the procedure that can be more successful once performed, and before irreversible fibrotic remodeling is established. The cut offs, based on right ventricular volume, are helpful for timing the first reoperation to treat severe PR [3, 4] but in case of prevalent stenosis it has been demonstrated to be insufficient [44]. Longitudinal and transversal strain allows a direct quantification of systolic and diastolic function of the right ventricle which may add value to the echocardiographic exam in decision making for reoperation of ToF. The cut off of -13% for global right ventricular longitudinal strain, in our preliminary data, seems to add value in selecting patients with adequate right ventricular functional reserves, who may respond to the PPV implant with consistent improvement of exercise tolerance and quality of life.

References

1. Liang XC, Cheung EW, Wong SJ, Cheung YF (2008) Impact of right ventricular volume overload on three-dimensional global left ventricular mechanical dyssynchrony after surgical repair of tetralogy of Fallot. Am J Cardiol 102:1731-1736
2. Gatzoulis MA, Balaji S, Webber SA et al (2000) Risk factors for arrhythmia and sudden cardiac death late after repair of tetralogy of Fallot: a multicentre study. Lancet 356:975-981
3. Therrien J, Provost Y, Merchant N et al (2005) Optimal timing for pulmonary valve replacement in adults after tetralogy of Fallot repair. Am J Cardiol 95:779-782

4. Frigiola A, Tsang V, Bull C et al (2008) Biventricular response after pulmonary valve replacement for right ventricular outflow tract dysfunction: is age a predictor of outcome? Circulation 118(14 Suppl):S182-190

5. Greutmann M, Tobler D, Biaggi P et al (2010) Echocardiography for assessment of right ventricular volumes revisited: a cardiac magnetic resonance comparison study in adults with repaired tetralogy of Fallot. J Am Soc Echocardiogr 23:905-911

6. van der Zwaan HB, Helbing WA, Boersma E et al (2010) Usefulness of real-time three-dimensional echocardiography to identify right ventricular dysfunction in patients with congenital heart disease. Am J Cardiol 106:843-850

7. van der Zwaan HB, Helbing WA, McGhie JS et al (2010) Clinical value of real-time three-dimensional echocardiography for right ventricular quantification in congenital heart disease: validation with cardiac magnetic resonance imaging. J Am Soc Echocardiogr 23:134-140

8. Greutmann M, Tobler D, Biaggi P et al (2010) Echocardiography for assessment of regional and global right ventricular systolic function in adults with repaired tetralogy of Fallot. Int J Cardiol [Epub ahead of print]

9. Kobayashi J, Nakano S, Matsuda H et al (1989) Quantitative evaluation of pulmonary regurgitation after repair of tetralogy of Fallot using real-time flow imaging system. Jpn Circ J 53:721-727

10. Williams RV, Minich LL, Shaddy RE et al (2002) Comparison of Doppler echocardiography with angiography for determining the severity of pulmonary regurgitation. Am J Cardiol 89:1438-1441

11. Silversides CK, Veldtman GR, Crossin J et al (2003) Pressure half-time predicts hemodynamically significant pulmonary regurgitation in adult patients with repaired tetralogy of fallot. J Am Soc Echocardiogr 16:1057-1062

12. Jhaveri RR, Saric M, Kronzon I (2010) Uncommon Doppler echocardiographic findings of severe pulmonic insufficiency. J Am Soc Echocardiogr 23:1071-1075

13. Gatzoulis MA, Elliott JT, Guru V et al (2000) Right and left ventricular systolic function late after repair of tetralogy of Fallot. Am J Cardiol 86:1352-1357

14. Munkhammar P, Cullen S, Jogi P et al (1998) Early age at repair prevents restrictive right ventricular (RV) physiology after surgery for tetralogy of Fallot (TOF): diastolic RV function after TOF repair in infancy. J Am Coll Cardiol 32:1083-1087

15. Gatzoulis MA, Clark AL, Cullen S et al (1995) Right ventricular diastolic function 15 to 35 years after repair of tetralogy of Fallot. Restrictive physiology predicts superior exercise performance. Circulation 91:1775-1781

16. Di Salvo G, Pacileo G, Rea A (2010) Transverse strain predicts exercise capacity in systemic right ventricle patients. Int J Cardiol 145:193-196

17. Lurz P, Gaudin R, Taylor AM, Bonhoeffer P (2009) Percutaneous pulmonary valve implantation. Semin Thorac Cardiovasc Surg Pediatr Card Surg Annu 2009:112-117

18. Schwerzmann M, Samman AM, Salehian O et al (2007) Comparison of echocardiographic and cardiac magnetic resonance imaging for assessing right ventricular function in adults with repaired tetralogy of fallot. Am J Cardiol 99:1593-1597

19. Lang RM, Bierig M, Devereux RB et al (2005) Recommendations for chamber quantification: a report from the American Society of Echocardiography's Guidelines and Standards Committee and the Chamber Quantification Writing Group, developed in conjunction with the European Association of Echocardiography, a branch of the European Society of Cardiology. J Am Soc Echocardiogr 18:1440-1463

20. Denslow S, Wiles HB (1998) Right ventricular volumes revisited: a simple model and simple formula for echocardiographic determination. J Am Soc Echocardiogr 11:864-873

21. Kelly NF, Platts DG, Burstow DJ (2010) Feasibility of pulmonary valve imaging using three-dimensional transthoracic echocardiography. J Am Soc Echocardiogr 23:1076-1080

22. Irvine T, Li XN, Rusk R (2000) Three dimensional colour Doppler echocardiography for the characterisation and quantification of cardiac flow events. Heart 84 Suppl 2:II2-6

23. Iriart X, Montaudon M, Lafitte S et al (2009) Right ventricle three-dimensional echography in corrected tetralogy of fallot: accuracy and variability. Eur J Echocardiogr 10:784-792

24. Khoo NS, Young A, Occleshaw C et al (2009) Assessments of right ventricular volume and function using three-dimensional echocardiography in older children and adults with congenital heart disease: comparison with cardiac magnetic resonance imaging. J Am Soc Echocardiogr 22:1279-1288

25. Shimada YJ, Shiota M, Siegel RJ, Shiota T (2010) Accuracy of right ventricular volumes and function determined by three-dimensional echocardiography in comparison with magnetic resonance imaging: a meta-analysis study. J Am Soc Echocardiogr 23:943-953

26. Kjaergaard J, Iversen KK, Akkan D (2009) Predictors of right ventricular function as measured by tricuspid annular plane systolic excursion in heart failure. Cardiovasc Ultrasound 7:51

27. Lopez-Candales A, Rajagopalan N, Saxena N et al (2006) Right ventricular systolic function is not the sole determinant of tricuspid annular motion. Am J Cardiol 98:973-977

28. Koestenberger M, Ravekes W, Everett AD et al (2009) Right ventricular function in infants, children and adolescents: reference values of the tricuspid annular plane systolic excursion (TAPSE) in 640 healthy patients and calculation of z score values. J Am Soc Echocardiogr 22:715 719

29. Nunez-Gil IJ, Rubio MD, Carton AJ et al (2011) Determination of normalized values of the tricuspid annular plane systolic excursion (TAPSE) in 405 Spanish children and adolescents. Rev Esp Cardiol 64:674-680

30. Tei C (1995) New non-invasive index for combined systolic and diastolic ventricular function. J Cardiol 26:135-136

31. Abd El Rahman MY, Abdul-Khaliq H, Vogel M et al (2002) Value of the new Doppler-derived myocardial performance index for the evaluation of right and left ventricular function following repair of tetralogy of fallot. Pediatr Cardiol 23:502-507

32. Yasuoka K, Harada K, Toyono M et al (2004) Tei index determined by tissue Doppler imaging in patients with pulmonary regurgitation after repair of tetralogy of Fallot. Pediatr Cardiol 25:131-136

33. Bussadori C, Moreo A, Di Donato M et al (2009) A new 2D-based method for myocardial velocity strain and strain rate quantification in a normal adult and paediatric population: assessment of reference values. Cardiovasc Ultrasound 7:8

34. Frigiola A, Redington AN, Cullen S, Vogel M (2004) Pulmonary regurgitation is an important determinant of right ventricular contractile dysfunction in patients with surgically repaired tetralogy of Fallot. Circulation 110(11 Suppl 1):II153-157

35. Weidemann F, Eyskens B, Mertens L et al (2002) Quantification of regional right and left ventricular function by ultrasonic strain rate and strain indexes after surgical repair of tetralogy of Fallot. Am J Cardiol 90:133-138

36. van der Hulst AE, Delgado V, Holman ER et al (2010) Relation of left ventricular twist and global strain with right ventricular dysfunction in patients after operative "correction" of tetralogy of fallot. Am J Cardiol 106:723-729

37. Hayabuchi Y, Sakata M, Ohnishi T, Kagami S (2011) A novel bilayer approach to ventricular septal deformation analysis by speckle tracking imaging in children with right ventricular overload. J Am Soc Echocardiogr 24:1205-1212

38. Bussadori C, Arcidiacono P, Saracino C et al (2011) Right and left ventricular strain and strain rate in young adults before and after percutaneous atrial septal defect closure. Echocardiography 28:730-737

39. Bussadori C, Chessa M, Negura D et al (2010) Echocardiography evaluation in GUCH patients. Pediatr Med Chir 32:247-255

40. Jategaonkar SR, Scholtz W, Butz T et al (2009) Two-dimensional strain and strain rate imaging of the right ventricle in adult patients before and after percutaneous closure of atrial septal defects. Eur J Echocardiogr 10:499-502

41. Kurotobi S, Taniguchi K, Sano T et al (2005) Determination of timing for reoperation in patients after right ventricular outflow reconstruction. Am J Cardiol 95:1344-1350

42. Kutty S, Deatsman SL, Russell D et al (2008) Pulmonary valve replacement improves but does not normalize right ventricular mechanics in repaired congenital heart disease: a comparative assessment using velocity vector imaging. J Am Soc Echocardiogr 21:1216-1221

43.   Moiduddin N, Asoh K, Slorach C et al (2009) Effect of transcatheter pulmonary valve im-
      plantation on short-term right ventricular function as determined by two-dimensional speck-
      le tracking strain and strain rate imaging. Am J Cardiol 104:862-867
44.   Castaldi B (2011) Percutaneous pulmonary valve implantation: feasibility, efficacy and im-
      pact on cardiac function. Doctoral Dissertation, Second University of Naples (Italy)
45.   McElhinney DB, Hellenbrand WE, Zahn EM et al (2010) Short- and medium-term outcomes
      after transcatheter pulmonary valve placement in the expanded multicenter US melody valve
      trial. Circulation 122:507-516

Timing for RVOT Management

9

Harald Kaemmerer, Andreas Eicken and John Hess

9.1 Introduction

The long-term survival and the overall outcome for patients after surgical repair of ToF are favorable [1, 2]. Nevertheless in many cases significant residues and sequelae persist or develop.

Moderate to severe pulmonary regurgitation (PR) is one of the most common complications. In the past, PR was regarded as a benign lesion, as many patients tolerate PR well for a considerable time. However, PR can also result in progressive right ventricular (RV) enlargement, RV-fibrosis and biventricular dysfunction [2–8]. Finally, in the fourth decade of life only 50% of all patients are free from cardiac symptoms [9].

However, even today quantification of PR is difficult and it is also challenging to decide which patient will benefit from pulmonary valve replacement (PVR). For these reasons indications and timing for PVR are still controversial issues.

9.2 Clinical and Functional Assessment

9.2.1 Patient History

Patients with preserved systolic RV-function are free of symptoms for years or even decades. However, it should be kept in mind that patients with congenital heart anomalies often underestimate their disability, due to the fact that they have adapted to it.

H. Kaemmerer (✉)
Department of Pediatric Cardiology and Congenital Heart Disease, German Heart Center,
Technical University of Munich, Munich, Germany
e-mail: kaemmerer@dhm.mhn.de

M. Chessa, A. Giamberti (eds.), *The Right Ventricle in Adults with Tetralogy of Fallot,*
© Springer-Verlag Italia 2012

In PR with significant degree, the compensatory mechanisms of the RV fail, the RV afterload increases, and the ejection fraction of the RV declines [10]. At that stage patients usually present with diminished exercise tolerance, fatigue, dyspnea on exertion, and sometimes with palpitations due to supraventricular or ventricular arrhythmias.

An impaired clinical status in long-term survivors after ToF repair is not only associated with the degree of PR: a low left ventricular ejection fraction is a strong, independent factor associated with impaired clinical status, perhaps by means of ventricular-ventricular interaction, where one ventricle influences the other adversely [11–13].

9.2.2   Physical Examination

Physical examination reveals a jugular venous pulse that is normal without right heart failure, or mild to moderate systemic venous pressure elevation with a prominent a-wave [14]. In tricuspid regurgitation, the jugular venous pressure may be elevated, showing a large v wave.

A parasternal lift from the right ventricle is palpable in almost all patients, while the left ventricular apical impulse is usually absent due to posterior displacement.

At the left upper sternal border a prominent main pulmonary artery impulse may be present.

On auscultation some adults have an early systolic pulmonary ejection sound, and a fourth heart sound. The aortic component of the second heart sound is loud, because of the anterior position of the aorta, while the pulmonary component of the widely and fixed split second heart sound is usually diminished in PR.

There is usually a spindle-shaped systolic murmur in the pulmonary area, indicating some degree of right ventricular outflow tract obstruction or pulmonary valve or pulmonary artery stenosis [15].

An isodynamic holosystolic murmur of tricuspid regurgitation, increasing its intensity after inspiration, may occur at the left lower parasternal border.

Pathognomonic for PR is a diastolic decrescendo murmur at the left upper parasternal border. The murmur starts immediately after the (diminished) pulmonary component of the second heart sound, and is medium to low pitched. The duration of the murmur is variable, depending on the degree of PR. With mild PR it is usually short, with moderate PR it is nearly holodiastolic, and, again shorter with severe PR [16]. As PR is associated with a low pulmonary artery pressure, the intensity of the murmur is usually low [17].

A third heart sound as well as hepatosplenomegaly, a pulsatile liver, ascites or peripheral edema may occur with right heart failure [14].

9.2.3 ECG

A right bundle branch block pattern is almost following ToF repair, even if no ventriculotomy has been performed [18]. There are only a few exceptions to this rule.

QRS duration may increase over years, often associated with greater right ventricular size. The greater the RV volume and mass are, the longer is the duration of the QRS-complex.

In particular, a progressive QRS duration > 180 ms may be a warning sign of ventricular arrhythmia and sudden death [19]. QRS duration of more than 180 ms had a 100% sensitivity for sustained VT and sudden death, while a QRS duration of less than 180 ms had a negative predictive value of 100% for these events [19].

The change in QRS duration over time (mean 3.5 ms/year) is an additional predictor of increased risk of sudden death [20].

The clinical relevance of these data for the individual, however, should be interpreted with caution. Some even believe that QRS prolongation is rather a marker of RV-dysfunction but not for sudden death.

QT dispersion or heart rate turbulence as an expression of an impaired cardiac autonomic nervous activity may be adjuvant methods of risk assessment [17, 21].

The ECG may also show right atrial enlargement (P-dextroatriale), right axis deviation, and right ventricular hypertrophy [15].

Atrial or ventricular arrhythmias may be present, and need further evaluation.

9.2.4 Chest X-ray

The cardiothoracic ratio (CTR) largely depends on the right ventricular volume load [15]. Depending on the amount of RV dilatation due to significant PR the CTR is usually increased to more than 0.55.

9.2.5 Echocardiography

Transthoracic echocardiographic (TTE) and Doppler assessment of the RV, pulmonary artery and PR is the first-line imaging modality in the follow-up of ToF-patients. In addition, residual RV outflow obstruction, pulmonary artery stenosis, residual shunts, and tricuspid regurgitation can be evaluated.

Because of the complex RV-geometry, the transthoracic echocardiographic evaluation of right ventricular volumes, function and mass has several limitations, and surrogate markers, such as fractional area shortening, tricuspid annular motion and tissue Doppler velocities, have to be applied [22].

Perhaps three-dimensional TTE will elude some limitations in the volumetric assessment of the RV at some point.

In patients with moderate to severe pulmonary regurgitation, color flow depicts a flow reversed blood flow from the right or left pulmonary artery to the RV body in diastole. However, doppler assessment may easily overestimate pulmonary regurgitation.

As the end-diastolic RV pressure is often only a few mmHg lower than the diastolic pulmonary artery pressure it can be difficult to reliably grade the severity of the PR [17]. In adults pulmonary pressure half-time of less than 100 milliseconds has been proposed as a good indicator of hemodynamically significant PR [23].

Some postoperative patients have a restrictive RV-function that is consistent with a lesser degree of pulmonary regurgitation. This type of diastolic dysfunction is marked by an antegrade diastolic flow in the pulmonary artery, and a flow reversal in the superior vena cava during atrial systole. The tricuspid E-wave deceleration time is short.

Even if a restrictive RV-hemodynamic is adverse in the early postoperative period, it has emerged as advantageous in the long term and may preclude RV-dilatation in spite of significant PR [24, 25].

9.2.6 Exercise Test

It is well known that PR after tetralogy repair may cause, besides malignant ventricular arrhythmia and sudden death [19, 26], reduced exercise performance [27-29].

Exercise studies with determination of maximum oxygen consumption and anaerobic threshold are helpful to assign symptomatology, objectively graduate exercise capacity, and to unmask exercise limitations secondary to PR. Exercise parameters are also important for an appropriate decision making on PVR in time.

9.2.7 Magnetic Resonance Imaging, Computed Tomography and Nuclear Cardiology

Cardiac Magnetic Resonance (CMR) is an ideal tool for serial assessment of RV-volumes and systolic function in the longitudinal follow-up after ToF-repair, providing good accuracy and reproducibility of not only important anatomic details of both ventricles, pulmonary arteries, and the aorta, but also functional data about right and left ventricular size, function and muscle mass, ventricular-ventricular interaction as well as flow and regurgitant volumes [7, 9, 13, 30].

Meanwhile CMR is regarded as the gold standard for the evaluation of RV-size and function as well as for the quantitative assessment of PR. Hereby the deficiency of older studies, with their lack of reproducible data regarding the severity of PR and RV-size and function, has been overcome. Age and gender have related reference values for right ventricular volumes and systolic function have been published [31].

A recent CMR-study determined that RV-dilatation and systolic RV-dysfunction or LV-dysfunction were independent predictors of major adverse clinical outcomes at a median of 21 years after ToF repair. High-risk CMR parameters in this study included a preoperative RV end-diastolic volume Z-score of 7 (corresponding to 172 cc/m2 in women, and 185 cc/m2 in men), or a global systolic dysfunction (ejection fraction < 45%) [32].

Modern computerized tomography (CT) provides data in patients with pacemakers, or other contraindications for MRI.

Nuclear cardiology studies can be used for the evaluation of RV-function and quantitative radionuclide flow studies reveal the amount of blood flow to each lung in patients with right or left pulmonary artery stenosis.

9.2.8 Cardiac Catheterization

The main purpose of cardiac catheterization in patients with PR is to determine ventricular physiology, right ventricular or pulmonary artery obstruction or residual shunts. It is particularly indicated if the hemodynamic status is not clarified by non-invasive procedures.

9.3 Treatment Options

There are no data indicating that medical treatment is able to slow the progression of PR. Currently no sufficient reliable data are available regarding the influence of selective pulmonary vasodilators on the outcome of patients with PR after ToF repair.

Pulmonary valve replacement is at present the only option to reduce RV-size and to improve RV-function in the long term.

Surgical or interventional replacement of the regurgitant PV can stop PR and may even reverse the progression of complications developed from PR, including RV-dysfunction and tricuspid regurgitation (Figs. 9.1, 9.2). It remains controversial, however, whether ventricular arrhythmias can be remediated [33]. Notably, in a large cohort of patients, late PVR alone for symptomatic PR and RV-dilation did not reduce the incidence of ventricular arrhythmias and sudden death [34].

Therefore at the time of PVR patients with known arrhythmias should be considered for intraoperative ablative treatment.

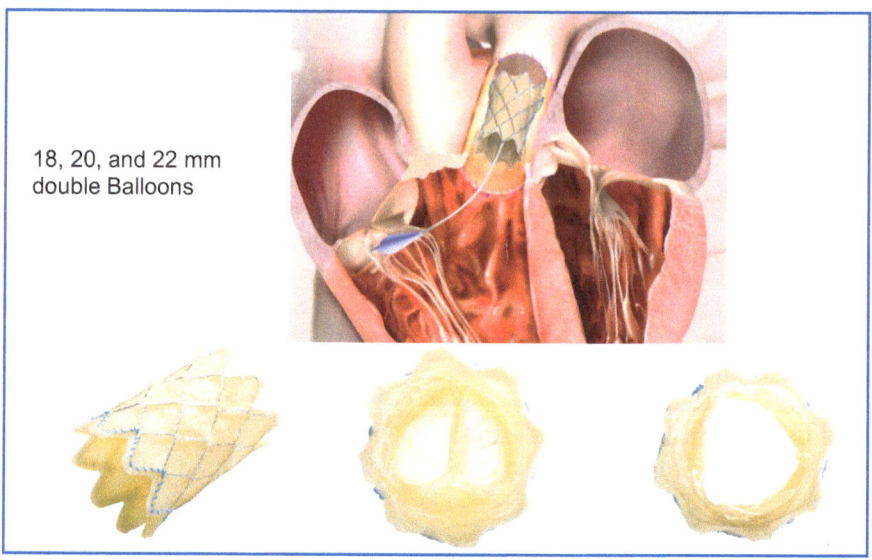

Fig. 9.1 The Melody valve is delivered over the superstiff guidewire on an 18, 20, or 22 mm double balloon into the right ventricular outflow tract. Courtesy of Medtronic Inc

18, 20, and 22 mm double Balloons

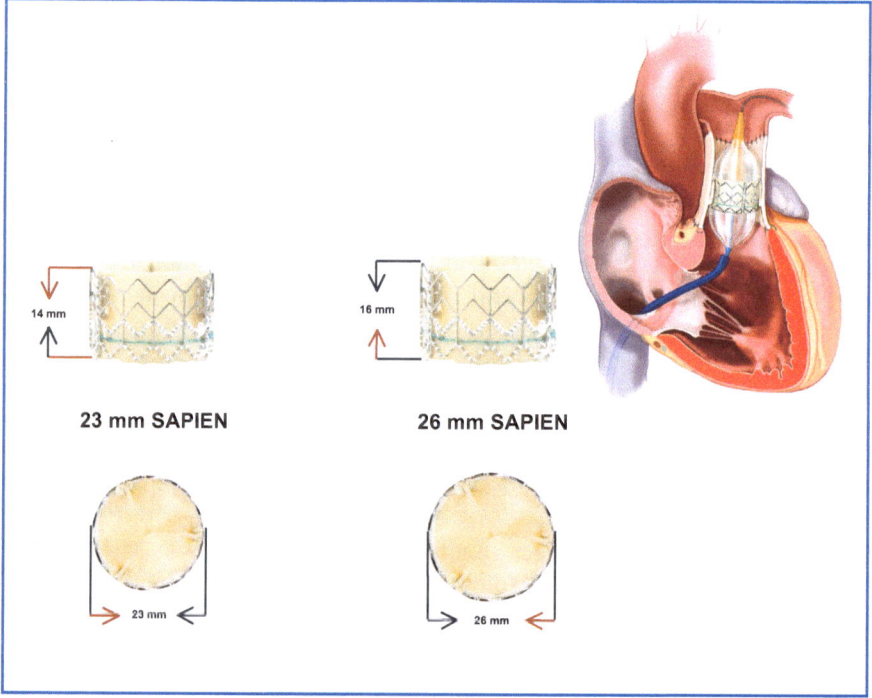

23 mm SAPIEN

26 mm SAPIEN

Fig. 9.2 The Sapien valve is available in two sizes (external diameter 23 and 26 mm, respectively). From Edwards Lifesciences with permission

9.4 Indication and Timing for Pulmonary Valve Replacement

In prevailing stenosis (RV systolic pressure > 60 mmHg, TR velocity > 3.5 m/s), selecting patients for therapy is relatively straightforward.

The treatment indication in patients with predominant pulmonary regurgitation or a combination of stenosis and regurgitation is not as simple. In fact most patients with right ventricular outflow tract dysfunction show a combination of obstruction and regurgitation [35].

The optimal timing of reoperation for significant PR after ToF repair is a matter of controversy given the limited runtime of the recently implanted prostheses and the risk of a further reoperation.

Currently, more and more experts recommend early surgery in these patients, before symptoms develop or RV-function has declined [36–38]. Today we believe that waiting for the patient to become symptomatic is not appropriate. In contrast, some believe that PVR should be performed only if RV-dysfunction is existent.

Unfortunately, currently no randomized controlled studies are available to help in the decision for timing therapy in the presence of significant pulmonary regurgitation.

An MRI study in adults with repaired ToF revealed a significant decrease in RV-volumes after PVR, while the RV systolic function remained unchanged. However, in patients with a RV end-diastolic volume > 170 ml/m^2 or a RV end-systolic volume > 85 ml/m^2 before PVR, the RV volumes did not return to normal after PVR [39].

However, in a study including younger patients with ToF and pulmonary regurgitation, RV remodeling after PVR could be shown at even higher right ventricular end diastolic (RVED) volume indices [37].

A threshold beyond which RV-function is unlikely to decrease to normal after surgery is difficult to specify at all. However, there seems to be an age- and volume index-dependent potential of the volume loaded right ventricle to remodel after adequate therapy for severe pulmonary regurgitation. Normalization of RV-volumes has been described when PVR was performed before the end-diastolic RV-volume reached 160 mL/m^2 or the end-systolic RV-volume reached 82 ml/m^2 [40].

Another group studied 71 consecutive patients (mean age 22 years, 72% ToF) pre and 1 year after PVR by cardiovascular MRI [41]. They concluded that treating patients with an end diastolic volume < 150 mL/m^2 leads to normalization of RV volumes, improvement in biventricular function, and submaximal exercise capability. Normalization of ventricular response to carbon dioxide production was most likely to occur when surgery was performed at an age </= 17.5 years.

To date, it is not clear whether a full normalization of RV-volumes is required for improving the outcome on a long-term course.

Altogether, even if the RV-volume is very high and RV dysfunction exists, PVR can reduce RV-size substantially, and improve RV-function, even if these

Table 9.1 Recommendations regarding pulmonary valve replacement in adults with previous ToF according to the current American, Canadian and European Guidelines

ACC/AHA Guidelines (2008) [42]	Pulmonary valve replacement is indicated for severe pulmonary regurgitation and symptoms or decreased exercise tolerance. Pulmonary valve replacement is reasonable in adults with previous ToF, severe pulmonary regurgitation, and any of the following: moderate to severe RV dysfunction; moderate to severe RV enlargement; development of symptomatic or sustained atrial and/or ventricular arrhythmias; moderate to severe TR.
Canadian Guidelines (2009) [43]	The following situations may warrant intervention following repair: free pulmonary regurgitation associated with progressive or moderate to severe RV enlargement (RV end-diastolic volume of greater than 170 ml/m^2), moderate to severe RV dysfunction, important tricuspid regurgitation atrial or ventricular arrhythmias, or symptoms such as deteriorating exercise performance.
European Guidelines (2010) [44]	PVRep should be performed in symptomatic patients with severe PR and/or stenosis (RV systolic pressure > 60 mmHg, TR velocity > 3.5m/s). PVRep should be considered in asymptomatic patients with severe PR and/or PS when at least one of the following criteria is present: decrease in objective exercise capacity; progressive RV dilation; progressive RV systolic dysfunction; progressive TR (at least moderate); RVOTO with RV systolic pressure > 80 mmHg (TR velocity > 4.3 m/s); sustained atrial/ventricular arrhythmias.

PR, pulmonary valve regurgitation; *PS*, pulmonary stenosis; *PVR*, pulmonary valve replacement; *RV*, right ventricular; *TR*, tricuspid valve regurgitation.

parameters may not decrease to the normal range. Apparently, regarding reverse remodeling, no threshold is present above which right ventricular volumes do not decrease after PVR.

One has to say constrictively, that given numbers should be interpreted with caution, as no mandatory regulations exist on how to measure ventricular volumes accurately, and therefore considerable differences have to be presumed!

In the last few years several international guidelines have been published focusing on the management of adults with ToF comprising certain discrepancies (Table 9.1). In addition, contemporary inclusion criteria for percutaneous pulmonary valve implantation (PPVI) as used at the German Heart Centre Munich are given in Table 9.2.

Table 9.2 Contemporary inclusion criteria for pulmonary valve replacement (PPVI) as used at the German Heart Centre Munich

German Heart Centre Munich (2011)	Increased RV-pressure (> 2/3 systemic pressure, Echo peak-gradient > 80 mmHg). Pulmonary regurgitation leading to a MRI-RVED-volume index > 150 ml/m², reduced and declining RV-function in cardiac MRI. A combination of stenosis and regurgitation with RV-dysfunction and dilatation. Symptomatic (?) patients with declining exercise tolerance (< 65% of normal). No clear lower age limit, looping of stiff delivery system is limited in small patients. Conduits or RV outflow tracts which can accommodate a covered stent to be dilated to at least 18 mm.

RV, right ventricle; *MRI*, magnetic resonance imaging.

All in all, PVR is at least indicated in patients developing symptoms due to severe pulmonary regurgitation, particularly if associated with substantial or progressive right ventricular dilatation, tricuspid regurgitation, and/or supraventricular or ventricular arrhythmias.

Finally, the long-term outcome of patients treated according to the current guidelines has to be evaluated.

References

1. Nollert G, Fischlein T, Bouterwek S et al (1997) Long-term survival in patients with repair of tetralogy of Fallot: 36-year follow-up of 490 survivors of the first year after surgical repair. J Am Coll Cardiol 30:1374-1383
2. Hickey EJ, Veldtman G, Bradley TJ et al (2009) Late risk of outcomes for adults with repaired tetralogy of Fallot from an inception cohort spanning four decades. Eur J Cardiothorac Surg 35:156-164
3. Graham TP Jr (2002) Management of pulmonary regurgitation after tetralogy of fallot repair. Curr Cardiol Rep 4:63-67
4. Redington AN (2006) Determinants and assessment of pulmonary regurgitation in tetralogy of Fallot: practice and pitfalls. Cardiol Clin 24:631-9, vii
5. Douzas B, Kilner PJ, Gatzoulis MA (2005) Pulmonary regurgitation: not a benign lesion. Eur Heart J 26:433-439
6. van Straten A, Vliegen HW, Hazekamp MG et al (2004) Right ventricular function after pulmonary valve replacement in patients with tetralogy of Fallot. Radiology 233:824-829
7. Babu-Narayan SV, Kilner PJ, Li W et al (2006) Ventricular fibrosis suggested by cardiovascular magnetic resonance in adults with repaired tetralogy of fallot and its relationship to adverse markers of clinical outcome. Circulation 113:405-413
8. Silka MJ, Hardy BG, Menashe VD, Morris CD (1998) A population-based prospective evaluation of risk of sudden cardiac death after operation for common congenital heart defects. J Am Coll Cardiol 32:245-251

9. Shimazaki Y, Blackstone EH, Kirklin JW (1984) The natural history of isolated congenital pulmonary valve incompetence: surgical implications. Thorac Cardiovasc Surg 32:257-259

10. Geva T (2006) Indications and timing of pulmonary valve replacement after tetralogy of Fallot repair. Semin Thorac Cardiovasc Surg Pediatr Card Surg Annu 11-22

11. Tobler D, Crean AM, Redington AN et al (2011) The left heart after pulmonary valve replacement in adults late after tetralogy of Fallot repair. Int J Cardiol [Epub ahead of print]

12. Geva T, Sandweiss BM, Gauvreau K et al (2004) Factors associated with impaired clinical status in long-term survivors of tetralogy of Fallot repair evaluated by magnetic resonance imaging. J Am Coll Cardiol 43:1068-1074

13. Davlouros PA, Kilner PJ, Hornung TS et al (2002) Right ventricular function in adults with repaired tetralogy of Fallot assessed with cardiovascular magnetic resonance imaging: detrimental role of right ventricular outflow aneurysms or akinesia and adverse right-to-left ventricular interaction. J Am Coll Cardiol 40:2044-2052

14. Ammash NM, Dearani JA, Burkhart HM, Connolly HM (2007) Pulmonary regurgitation after tetralogy of Fallot repair: clinical features, sequelae, and timing of pulmonary valve replacement. Congenit Heart Dis 2:386-403

15. Perloff JK (2003) Clinical Recognition of Congenital Heart Disease, 5 edn. Saunders, Philadelphia, pp 348-382

16. Perloff JK (2009) Physical examination of heart and circulation. PMPH USA Ltd, Shelton, pp 205-208

17. Bashore TM (2007) Adult congenital heart disease: right ventricular outflow tract lesions. Circulation 115:1933-1947

18. Horowitz LN, Simson MB, Spear JF et al (1979) The mechanism of apparent right bundle branch block after transatrial repair of tetralogy of Fallot. Circulation 59:1241-1252

19. Gatzoulis MA, Till JA, Somerville J, Redington AN (1995) Mechanoelectrical interaction in tetralogy of Fallot. QRS prolongation relates to right ventricular size and predicts malignant ventricular arrhythmias and sudden death. Circulation 92:231-237

20. Steeds RP, Oakley D (2004) Predicting late sudden death from ventricular arrhythmia in adults following surgical repair of tetralogy of Fallot. QJM 97:7-13

21. Lammers A, Kaemmerer H, Hollweck R et al (2006) Impaired cardiac autonomic nervous activity predicts sudden cardiac death in patients with operated and unoperated congenital cardiac disease. J Thorac Cardiovasc Surg 132:647-655

22. Lang RM, Bierig M, Devereux RB et al (2005) Recommendations for chamber quantification: a report from the American Society of Echocardiography's Guidelines and Standards Committee and the Chamber Quantification Writing Group, developed in conjunction with the European Association of Echocardiography, a branch of the European Society of Cardiology. J Am Soc Echocardiogr 18:1440-1463

23. Silversides CK, Veldtman GR, Crossin J et al (2003) Pressure half-time predicts hemodynamically significant pulmonary regurgitation in adult patients with repaired tetralogy of fallot. J Am Soc Echocardiogr 16:1057-1062

24. Lu JC, Cotts TB, Agarwal PP et al (2010) Relation of right ventricular dilation, age of repair, and restrictive right ventricular physiology with patient-reported quality of life in adolescents and adults with repaired tetralogy of fallot. Am J Cardiol 106:1798-1802

25. Gatzoulis MA, Clark AL, Cullen S (1995) Right ventricular diastolic function 15 to 35 years after repair of tetralogy of Fallot. Restrictive physiology predicts superior exercise performance. Circulation 91:1775-1781

26. Marie PY, Marcon F, Brunotte F et al (1992) Right ventricular overload and induced sustained ventricular tachycardia in operatively "repaired" tetralogy of Fallot. Am J Cardiol 69:785-789

27. Carvalho JS, Shinebourne EA, Busst C (1992) Exercise capacity after complete repair of tetralogy of Fallot: deleterious effects of residual pulmonary regurgitation. Br Heart J 67:470-473

28. Wessel HU, Cunningham WJ, Paul MH et al (1980) Exercise performance in tetralogy of Fallot after intracardiac repair. J Thorac Cardiovasc Surg 80:582-593

29. Kang IS, Redington AN, Benson LN et al (2003) Differential regurgitation in branch pulmonary

arteries after repair of tetralogy of Fallot: a phase-contrast cine magnetic resonance study. Circulation 107:2938-2943

30. Kilner PJ, Geva T, Kaemmerer H et al (2010) Recommendations for cardiovascular magnetic resonance in adults with congenital heart disease from the respective working groups of the European Society of Cardiology. Eur Heart J 31:794-805

31. Maceira AM, Prasad SK, Khan M, Pennell DJ (2006) Reference right ventricular systolic and diastolic function normalized to age, gender and body surface area from steady-state free precession cardiovascular magnetic resonance. Eur Heart J 27:2879-2888

32. Knauth AL, Gauvreau K, Powell AJ et al (2008) Ventricular size and function assessed by cardiac MRI predict major adverse clinical outcomes late after tetralogy of Fallot repair. Heart 94:211-216

33. Therrien J, Siu SC, Harris L et al (2001) Impact of pulmonary valve replacement on arrhythmia propensity late after repair of tetralogy of Fallot. Circulation 103:2489-2494

34. Harrild DM, Berul CI, Cecchin F et al (2009) Pulmonary valve replacement in tetralogy of Fallot: impact on survival and ventricular tachycardia. Circulation 119:445-451

35. Eicken A, Ewert P, Hager A et al (2011) Percutaneous pulmonary valve implantation: two-centre experience with more than 100 patients. Eur Heart J 32:1260-1265

36. Apitz C, Webb GD, Redington AN (2009) Tetralogy of Fallot. Lancet 374:1462-1471

37. Buechel ER, Dave HH, Kellenberger CJ et al (2005) Remodelling of the right ventricle after early pulmonary valve replacement in children with repaired tetralogy of Fallot: assessment by cardiovascular magnetic resonance. Eur Heart J 26:2721-2727

38. Henkens IR, van Straten A, Schalij MJ et al (2007) Predicting outcome of pulmonary valve replacement in adult tetralogy of Fallot patients. Ann Thorac Surg 83:907-911

39. Therrien J, Provost Y, Merchant N (2005) Optimal timing for pulmonary valve replacement in adults after tetralogy of Fallot repair. Am J Cardiol 95:779-782

40. Oosterhof T, van Straten A, Vliegen HW et al (2007) Preoperative thresholds for pulmonary valve replacement in patients with corrected tetralogy of Fallot using cardiovascular magnetic resonance. Circulation 116:545-551

41. Frigiola A, Tsang V, Bull C et al (2008) Biventricular response after pulmonary valve replacement for right ventricular outflow tract dysfunction: is age a predictor of outcome? Circulation 118(14 Suppl):S182-190

42. Warnes CA, Williams RG, Bashore TM et al (2008) ACC/AHA 2008 Guidelines for the management of adults with congenital heart disease: a report of the American College of Cardiology/American Heart Association Task Force on Practice Guidelines (writing committee to develop guidelines on the management of adults with congenital heart disease). Circulation 118:e714-833

43. Silversides CK, Kiess M, Beauchesne L et al (2010) Canadian Cardiovascular Society 2009 Consensus Conference on the management of adults with congenital heart disease: outflow tract obstruction, coarctation of the aorta, tetralogy of Fallot, Ebstein anomaly and Marfan's syndrome. Can J Cardiol 26:e80-97

44. Baumgartner H, Bonhoeffer P, De Groot NM et al (2010) ESC Guidelines for the management of grown-up congenital heart disease (new version 2010). Eur Heart J 31:2915-2957

Percutaneous Pulmonary Valve

10

Mark S. Turner, Mario Carminati and Philipp Bonhoeffer

Tetralogy of Fallot (ToF) and its surgical treatment frequently lead to dysfunction of the pulmonary valve. A common surgical approach to this is to implant a right ventricle to pulmonary artery valved conduit. Many conduits are available and their nature is important when considering a transcatheter valve. Pulmonary or aortic homografts (human donor valves) have been successfully used as a right ventricle to pulmonary artery conduit [1]. These conduits can fail causing progressive stenosis, or regurgitation, which can present at an early stage. Homografts are prone to calcification as well as endocarditis. Other conduits have been used including pericardial valves mounted in a prosthetic tube, such as a Hancock conduit (porcine) and a valved conduit of bovine jugular vein (Contegra). When a conduit is not needed some surgeons use stented bioprosthetic valves with pericardial leaflets to achieve a competent pulmonary valve [2].

Patients with failing conduits have necessarily had at least one open surgical procedure, to implant the conduit. However, many patients will have had multiple operations, and as the number of operations increases, so does the surgical risk. In order to reduce the number of operations, we developed the first percutaneous valve that was first implanted in a human on 12th September 2000 in Paris [3]. This valve, with some modification, is now commercially available as the Melody valve by Medtronic and has provided the majority of data in this field.

The Melody valve is a length of bovine jugular vein containing a venous valve, sutured into a 34 mm platinum iridium Cheatham Platinum (CP) stent, producing a covered stent with the valve leaflets near its proximal end (Fig. 10.1). The thin compliant leaflets of the venous valve pack more easily into a delivery catheter and the geometric structure of the leaflets enable them to

M.S. Turner (✉)
Department of Cardiology, Bristol Heart Institute, Bristol, UK
e-mail: markturner45@hotmail.com

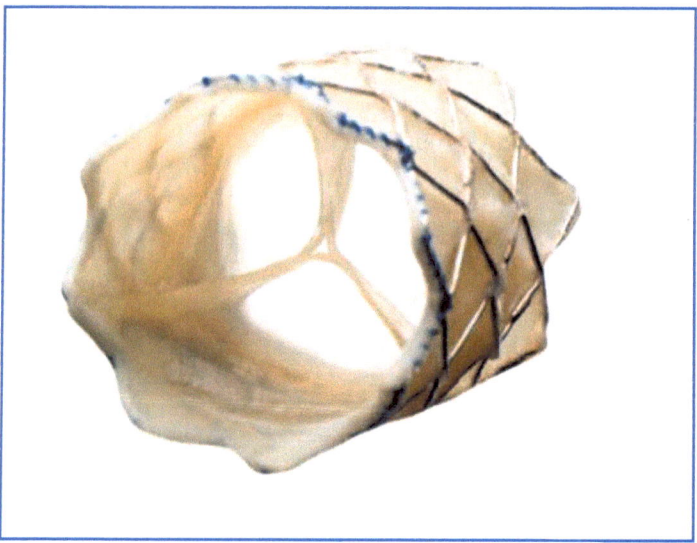

Fig. 10.1 A Melody valve viewed from the distal end, looking down onto the three leaflets. The Platinum stent can be seen and the thinned vein wall can be appreciated by the translucency allowing the stent frame to be seen through it

work at a wide range of diameters and shapes (as a venous valve has to in a vein), whereas pericardial tissue prosthetic valves function best at their design size and shape. Failing conduits are rarely circular and have complex shapes and stenoses, but the Melody valve remains competent in different sizes and geometries [4]. The Edwards-Sapien bovine pericardial valve is now available for use in the pulmonary position, having been developed for the aortic valve indication. This is a stent with a pericardial valve mounted within it, necessitating expansion to the design size and shape. The Edwards Sapien Valve finds its major indication in the treatment of larger conduits up to 25 mm, overcoming the size limitation of the Melody valve at 22 mm.

The jugular vein surrounding the valve is thinned by removing external layers prior to being sutured into the stent, and coupled with the thin venous valve leaflets, allows it to be packed into a relatively small diameter catheter. Fixation relies on the stent being well applied to the wall of the conduit, and by delivering the valve with its center in a stenosis, with distal and proximal ends flaring a little. The delivery system is flexible enough to track around the curves of the right heart and robust enough to be able to cross calcified conduits. It also keeps the valve covered until in position in the conduit, preventing dislodgement of the stent from the balloon. Once in position the stent can be inflated using the balloon in balloon (BIB) system. Delivery systems of 18 mm, 20 mm and 22 mm balloon sizes are available, 22 mm being the maximum diameter at which the bovine jugular valve remains competent.

Initial experience demonstrated the Melody valve to be a safe and effective alternative to surgical conduit replacement in a range of congenital heart lesions [4]. ToF patients were well represented, but the experience also includes patients with a range of congenital heart malformations such as aortic stenosis patients treated with the Ross operation and Transposition treated by a Rastelli operation. Clinical efficacy was shown in studies of many relevant parameters describing clinical end points such as exercise capacity and symptoms and catheter and imaging-based assessments of right ventricular performance and hemodynamics [5-7].

Complications did occur, but overall the Melody procedure has a lower mortality than open surgical replacement of the pulmonary valve. The Central Cardiac Audit Database in England captures nearly all surgical valve replacements and the mortality for open PVR is usually 1–2% each year, and thus similar to published surgical series [1]. Melody implantation carries a mortality of around 0.3% or less. Combining the data from the London, U.S. and German experience papers, major complications are homograft rupture 1.3%, coronary compression 0.8%, perforation of a distal pulmonary artery 1%, device dislodgement/embolization 0.5%, damage to tricuspid valve 0.5% and obstruction of the main pulmonary artery 0.5%. No other complication was reported to be greater than or equal to 0.5%.

Homograft rupture and coronary compression are the most feared complications. Meticulous assessment of the patient prior to implantation should be able to evaluate the risk of coronary compression. Furthermore, in patients judged to be at risk, the conduit should be dilated with a balloon to the planned size with a simultaneous coronary angiogram, prior to pre-stenting to avoid this complication [8]. Coronary stenting is unlikely to hold a coronary open against the force of a large stent and if coronary compression occurs urgent surgical removal of the stent is likely to be needed.

Homograft rupture may be treated by surgery or covered stenting, but the bleeding may also stop with reversal of heparin. Autotransfusion using a cell saver has been used to good effect. Some patients may be candidates for transplantation later in life so avoiding donor blood transfusion is desirable. Reducing the number of sternotomies by using percutaneous approaches may also reduce the risk of heart transplantation if needed later.

Early problems with "hammocking", where the walls of the vein were sucked inwards by the Bernoulli effect from the blood flow creating obstruction, were dealt with by additional suturing of the vein to the stent. Fractures of the CP stent were also seen with a rate of 21% in the London experience [9]. The right ventricular outflow tract is a hostile environment for rigid metallic stents where calcification of the conduit and motion of the muscle in the RV outflow tract can lead to metal fatigue and consequent stent fracture. Of the 21% with stent fractures, many of these did not have any clinical consequence if the fractures did not affect stent integrity, but severe fractures have led to embolization into the lungs on one occasion and restenosis in others. Risk factors for fracture were; "native" outflow tract (meaning no conduit), absence of

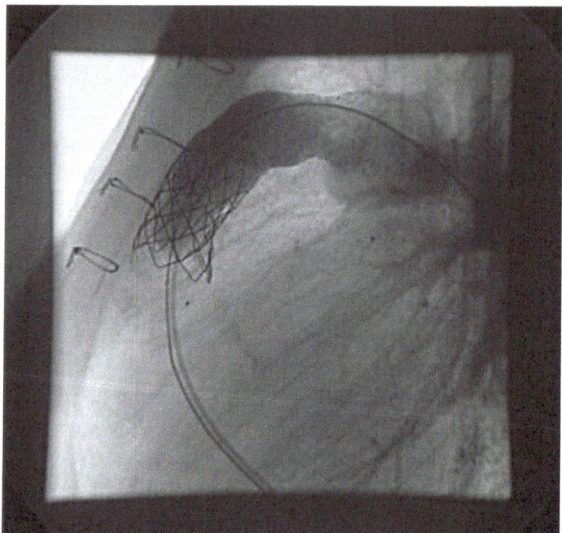

Fig. 10.2 A Melody valve implanted in a 13 year old boy with pulmonary atresia and three previous sternotomies. The conduit has been extensively pre-stented with LD Max stents

calcification and recoil of the stent when the balloon was deflated [10]. Reintervention with a second percutaneous valve is however a feasible treatment option for this complication [11]. Fractures have been improved by a change in implantation technique; current practice is to implant one or more stents within the conduit until it is prepared for the valve [12]. Acquiring an X-ray cine angiogram at the moment the pre-stent balloon deflation can determine if there is any recoil of the stent, in which case a further stent can strengthen the segment for Melody implantation. The recently published German results, show a much improved stent fracture rate of only 5%, which is likely to be due to pre-stenting [7]. Pre-stenting can also provide additional stability, particularly if the conduit is near the maximum size of the Melody valve stent, or if the circumference of the conduit contains potentially distensible areas. For these reasons virtually all Melody implants are now performed into a pre-stented conduit. The figures show two examples of pre-stented conduits (Figs. 10.2 and 10.3), and one of the Melody being implanted without pre-stenting into a stented surgical tissue valve (Fig. 10.4).

Whilst many of these patients had ToF as their primary congenital malformation, the majority of ToF patients with a transannular patch have regurgitation with little obstruction and therefore the observations made about the right ventricle in the Melody cohort cannot be extrapolated to all ToF patients with a transannular patch, who have never had a conduit. Despite this limitation, as well as providing a less invasive and clinically effective technique for treating patients with failing conduits, the Melody procedure provides a superb model for studying the effects of improving pulmonary valve function on the right ventricle, without the confounding effects of opening the chest, disturbing the

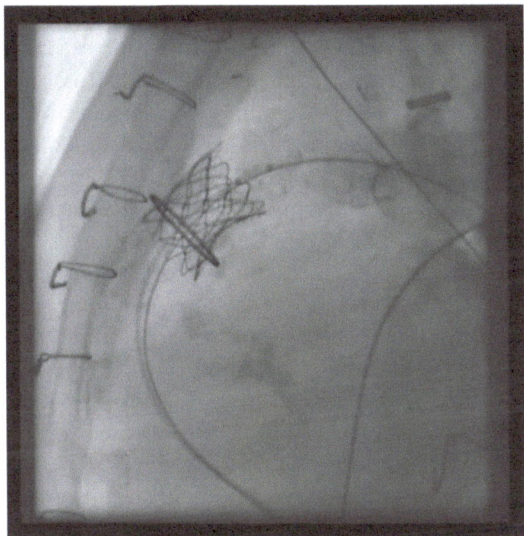

Fig. 10.3 A Melody valve implanted into a Hancock conduit, which was pre-stented. Note the previous pulmonary artery stent

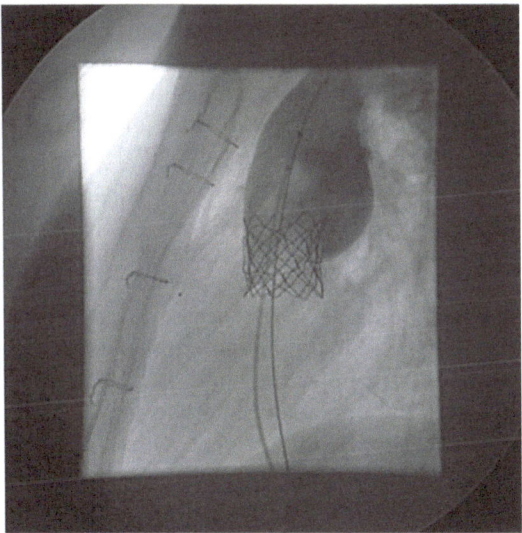

Fig. 10.4 This patient had undergone surgical replacement of the pulmonary valve with a 23 mm Perimount pericardial valve prosthesis, which became severely stenotic. A Melody was implanted without pre-stenting, as the valve ring was not thought to pose a fracture risk. The gradient was successfully reduced and there have been no complications in follow up

pericardium and subjecting the right ventricle to the detrimental effects of cardiopulmonary bypass.

The Melody cohort are selected both by having a conduit and also by having some degree of stenosis in the RVOT, as patients with an outflow tract greater than 22 mm are excluded. The majority of the data on right ventricular function comes from our London experience. Coats et al. [5] reported on 18 patients with severe conduit stenosis (echo gradient > 50mmHg) treated with Melody. Six patients had ToF and four had pulmonary atresia with a VSD as their initial diagnosis, with the remainder being Transposition, post-Ross and Truncus. All but one patient had a homograft. The Melody was successful in reducing catheter gradients from 51.4 to 21.7 mmHg. The clinical outcomes were excellent with improved exercise capacity.

Magnetic resonance imaging (MRI) studies pre-procedure and at a mean of 6 days post-procedure, showed a reduction in RV end diastolic volumes and increased ejection fraction and stroke volume. Interestingly, reduction in RV volume was accompanied by an increase in left ventricular volume. The authors offered three explanations for these observations. Firstly, improved filling of the left ventricle due to increased pulmonary blood flow as a consequence of the increased stroke volume of the right ventricle was proposed.

Secondly, rather than improved pulmonary blood flow causing the improvement in filling, an alternative hypothesis is that the reduced RV volume and reduced RV end diastolic pressure relieved external constraint on the left ventricle. Diastolic ventricular interaction has long been recognized as a feature of left ventricular failure and acute pulmonary embolus, where the right ventricle and pericardium impede left ventricular filling [13, 14]. In these conditions the pericardium reaches its elastic limit, whereby increased stretch leads to an increasing pericardial pressure. As true filling pressure of the left ventricle is the pressure across the myocardium, this equates to left atrial pressure minus the pericardial pressure (which is usually assumed to be the same as the right ventricular end diastolic pressure). Thus if the right ventricle reduces in size and the right ventricular end diastolic pressure (RVEDP) falls, the pericardial pressure will fall and the true filling pressure of the left ventricle will increase, even if the left atrial pressure remains the same.

Thirdly the possibility of improved ventricular contractility was proposed, but immediately rejected by the authors as the tissue Doppler component of their study showed no change in iso-volumic acceleration and the improved tricuspid annulus systolic wave was only transiently increased, thus there was no load independent or sustained evidence of improved contractility [5].

Further evidence to support the diastolic interaction hypothesis was found by Lurz et al. [15], who studied septal motion and left ventricular filling by MRI in 20 consecutive patients (the majority having had ToF), with predominant conduit stenosis, before and after Melody implantation. This study showed that the septal interaction was decreased by the Melody implantation and the septal position was improved such that it no longer moved towards the left ventricle. This normalized geometry of the septum was associated with improved early filling of the left ventricle and this feature was felt to be responsible for the clinical improvement. Furthermore they showed a reduced interventricular mechanical delay between the left and right ventricles, measured by echocardiography. The time to onset of pulmonary flow did not appear to be shortened, but the filling of the right ventricle started earlier, presumably due to a more rapid ejection phase or a lower RVEDP allowing earlier onset of filling. Dysynchrony has also been proposed to occur with exercise in ToF patients [16], and modification of synchrony can alter diastolic interaction in left heart failure [17]. Whatever the mechanisms, treating pulmonary valve dysfunction not only improves right ventricular volumes, but it can also improve left ventricular performance [18]. This may also help to explain the cause of left ventricular dysfunction late after ToF repair. The evidence that left ventricular dysfunction in ToF is associated with sudden death [19] has led to the proposal that early treatment of pulmonary valve dysfunction is likely to prevent many of the problems previously observed in these patients. However, it has also been observed that younger patients are more likely to normalize their right ventricular function after valve implantation, again supporting the argument for earlier intervention to preserve the right ventricle [20].

Transcatheter treatments are generally more acceptable to patients and their parents than surgery, which may lead to earlier treatment of valve dysfunction. As further developments in transcatheter valve technology emerge, we anticipate an increasing acceptance of earlier treatment of asymptomatic individuals leading to reductions in late complications of ToF and other cardiac malformations affecting the pulmonary valve. A self-expanding valve to treat pulmonary regurgitation in large outflow tracts has already been reported [21], and the use of pre-stenting to allow treatment of some patients without conduits with balloon expandable valved stents is gaining momentum. As a consequence of these advances, it is possible to envisage a time in the near future where percutaneous valve replacement may be available for a majority of patients with pulmonary valve dysfunction, which will hopefully lead to preservation of the right ventricular function in these patients.

References

1. Van de Woestijne PC, Mokhles MM, de Long PL et al (2011) Right ventricular outflow tract reconstruction with an allograft conduit in patients after tetralogy of Fallot correction: long-term follow-up. Ann Thorac Surg 92:161-166
2. Lee C, Park CS, Lee CH, Kwak JG et al (2011) Durability of bioprosthetic valves in the pulmonary poisiton: long-term follow up of 181 implants in patients with congenital heart disease. J Thorac Cardiovasc Surg 142:351-358
3. Bonhoeffer P, Boudjemline Y, Saliba Z et al (2000) Percutaneous replacement of pulmonary valve in the right ventricle to pulmonary artery prosthetic conduit with valve dysfunction. Lancet 356:1403-1405
4. Khambadkone S, Coats L, Taylor A et al (2005) Percutaneous pulmonary valve implantation in humans: results in 59 consecutive patients. Circulation 112:1189-1197
5. Coats L, Khambadkone S, Derrick G et al (2006) Physiological and clinical consequences of relief of right ventricular outflow tract obstruction late after repair of congenital heart defects. Circulation 113:2037-2044
6. Coats L, Khambadkone S, Derrick G et al (2007) Physiological consequences of percutaneous pulmonary valve replacement; the different behaviour of volume and pressure-overloaded ventricles. Eur Heart J 28:1886-1893
7. Eicken A, Ewert P, Hager A et al (2011) Percutaneous pulmonary valve implantation: two centre experience of over 100 patients. Eur Heart J 32:1260-1265

8. Sridharan S, Coats L, Khambadkone S et al (2006) Transcatheter right ventricular outflow tract intervention: The risk to the coronary circulation. Circulation 113:e934-935

9. Nordmeyer J, Khambadkone S, Coats L et al (2007) Risk stratification, systematic classification, and anticipatory management strategies for stent fracture after percutaneous pulmonary valve implantation. Circulation 115:1392-1397

10. Schievano S, Petrini L, Migliavacca F et al (2007) Finite element analysis of stent deployment: understanding stent fractures in percutaneous pulmonary valve implantation. J Interv Cardiol 20:546-554

11. Nordmeyer J, Coats L, Lurz P et al (2008) Percutaneous pulmonary valve-in-valve implantation: a successful treatment concept for early device failure. Eur Heart J 29:810-815

12. Nordmeyer J, Lurz P, Khambadkone S et al (2011) Pre-stenting with bare metal stent before percutaneous pulmonary valve implantation: acute and 1-year outcomes. Heart 97:118-123

13. Atherton JJ, Moore TD, Lele SS et al (1997) Diastolic ventricular interaction in chronic heart failure. Lancet 349:1720-1724

14. Morris-Thurgood JA, Frenneaux MP (2000) Diastolic ventricular interaction and ventricular diastolic filling. Heart Fail Rev 5:307-323

15. Lurz P, Puranik R, Nordmeyer J (2009) Improvement in left ventricular filling properties after relief of right ventricle to pulmonary artery conduit obstruction: contribution of septal motion and interventricular mechanical delay. Eur Heart J 30:2266-2274

16. Tobler D, Crean AM, Redington AN et al (2011) The left heart after pulmonary valve replacement in adults late after tetralogy of Fallot repair. Int J Cardiol [Epub ahead of print]

17. Roche SL, Grosse-Wortmann L, Redington AN et al (2010) Exercise induces biventricular mechanical dyssynchrony in children with repaired tetralogy of Fallot. Heart 96:2010-2015

18. Bleasdale RA, Turner MS, Mumford CE et al (2004) Left ventricular pacing minimizes diastolic ventricular interaction, allowing improved preload-dependent systolic performance. Circulation 110:2395-2400

19. Ghai A, Silversides C, Harris L et al (2002) Left ventricular dysfunction is a risk factor for sudden cardiac death in adults late after repair of tetralogy of Fallot. J Am Coll Cardiol 40:1675-1680

20. Frigiola A, Tsang V, Bull C et al (2008) Biventricular response after pulmonary valve replacement for right ventricular outflow tract dysfunction: is age a predictor of outcome? Circulation 118:S182-190

21. Schievano S, Taylor AM, Capelli C et al (2010) First-in-man implantation of a novel percutaneous valve: a new approach to medical device development. Euro Intervention 5:745-750

Other Transcatheter Procedures

11

Massimo Chessa and Gianfranco Butera

11.1 Introduction

The interventional approach to the management of congenital heart disease (CHD) in the adult population is becoming increasingly recognized as the preferred treatment option for a wide number of congenital cardiac conditions [1]. Many of the catheter interventional techniques have been effective in the management of subjects pre- and post surgical repair of ToF.

A recent study showed that the overall survival rate after complete repair of ToF at 10, 20 and 25 years was 94.8%, 92.8% and 92.8%, respectively [2]. Half of survivors may undergo a reoperation 30 years after correction [3–5]. There are different situations requiring consideration for reintervention: residual atrial septal defects (ASD) or ventricular septal defects (VSD) with a shunt, residual patent arterial shunts leading to left ventricular volume overload, residual pulmonary valvular/supravalvular stenosis, residual pulmonary branch artery stenosis, pulmonary valve regurgitation, aortic valve regurgitation, progressive aortic root enlargement.

In the previous chapters the surgical or transcatheter management of some of these different sequelae were treated.

In this chapter, we will discuss the management of residual ventricular septal defects and pulmonary branch artery stenosis in the catheterization laboratory.

M. Chessa (✉)
IRCCS Policlinico San Donato, Pediatric and Adult Congenital Heart Center,
San Donato Milanese (Mi), Italy
e-mail: massichessa@yahoo.it

M. Chessa, A. Giamberti (eds.), *The Right Ventricle in Adults with Tetralogy of Fallot,*
© Springer-Verlag Italia 2012

11.2   Pulmonary Branch Artery Stenosis

A recent study by Park et al. [6] reported an incidence of pulmonary branch artery stenosis of 17.9%. Authors found that stenosis of the pulmonary branch artery occurred at the level of left pulmonary artery (LPA) in 64.6% of patients, the right pulmonary artery (RPA) was involved in 9.4%, while both were involved pulmonary arteries in 26%.

Stenosis may be discrete or associated with long segment hypoplasia, and may be congenital or secondary to a previous surgical procedure. Post surgical stenosis is most commonly due to scar formation, especially at the site of a shunt, at the edges of a patch arterioplasty, or at the anastomotic sites of previous unifocalized vessels.

Obstruction within the pulmonary arterial tree can result in elevated right ventricular pressures and potentially worsen pulmonary insufficiency in patients with repaired ToF. This can lead to ventricular dysfunction, ultimately increasing the risk of ventricular arrhythmias and sudden death [7]. Ideally, interventions should take place prior to development of signs or symptoms from chronic pulmonary obstruction. Universally accepted indications for intervention include symptoms, iso- or supra-systemic right ventricular pressure or dysfunction, and significant differential pulmonary perfusion. Non invasive imaging, such as echocardiograms and magnetic resonance imaging (MRI) are useful for monitoring patients with known or suspected disease, and can be used to define the ideal timing for interventions in absence of symptoms.

Relief of the stenosis and reduction of the pressure gradient can be obtained by surgery, if the stenosis is proximal; however if the stenosis is located in a peripheral area of the lungs, transcatheter balloon dilation is a therapeutic option.

In 1983, Lock et al. [8] first described balloon dilation angioplasty of branch pulmonary stenosis in a series of seven patients. Balloon angioplasty for pulmonary artery stenosis is not uniformly successful, with several reports suggesting an acute success rate in the range of only 50%, with clinical management favorably influenced in only 35% of patients. It was clear from the beginning that stenotic lesions in pulmonary arteries were unpredictable, and variable in their response to balloon dilation. The introduction of high-pressure balloons improved the results of simple angioplasty [9], but a subset of vessels remained resistant to therapy, with recoil of the stenotic artery after dilation [10]. In the late 1980s, therefore, Mullins et al. [11] using a canine model, assessed the potential role of stents in the relief of obstructed pulmonary arteries; since then different stents have become available on the market, but the ideal stent for congenital and post operative lesions is not available.

Procedures are generally performed under general anesthesia with oro-tracheal intubation. Arterial monitoring line is suggested; one or two femoral (if possible) venous sheaths are currently placed. We usually prefer to insert a Mullins long sheath that can be used for both dilatation/stent placement and angiograms before, during and after the procedure. After a complete right

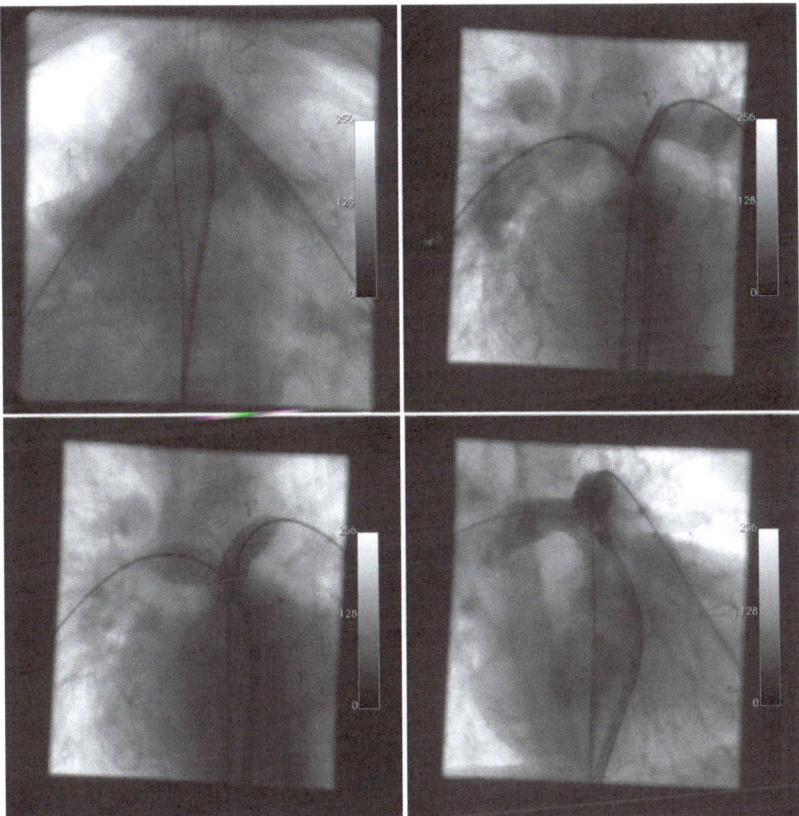

Fig. 11.1 Proximal bilateral pulmonary artery stenosis and moderate hypoplasia. Pulmonary artery angiography with caudal and left anterior oblique angulation (*upper left*); pulmonary artery angiography with cranial and left anterior oblique angulation showing two stent-balloon assembly at the origin of the two pulmonary arteries (*upper right*); simultaneous balloon inflation (*bottom left*); angiography showing the two stents in place with significant increase of vessel diameter (*bottom right*)

heart catheterization the catheter is advanced to the desired lung.

Angiographic assessment is best done with the most selective catheter position possible. It is absolutely essential to have excellent wire support for placement of a dilating balloon or stents. The initial suggested balloon diameter needs to be 3–3.5 times the diameter of the stenosis to be effective. High pressure balloons may be used for larger vessels. The use of cutting balloons (balloons with three or four microtome blades fastened along the length of the balloon), is currently limited and applicable primarily to small vessels.

If the angioplasty is not effective and the desired effect is not achieved, the next option is stent implantation. In adult patients we prefer stenting as the primary treatment for stenotic vessels, because it prevents most of the vessel elastic recoil (Figs. 11.1–11.3). The best stent used is the shortest that can be dilat-

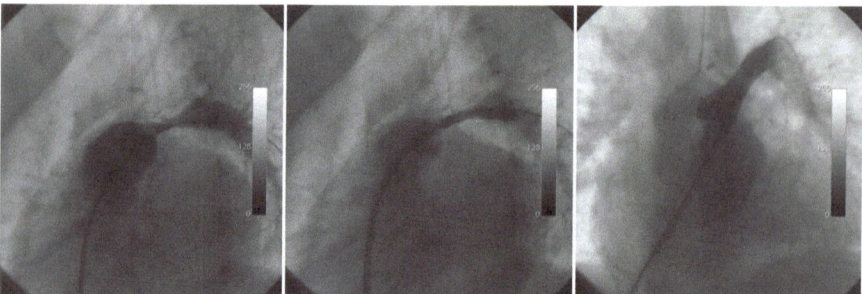

Fig. 11.2 Left pulmonary artery stenosis in a patient operated on for ToF. Left pulmonary angiography in left anterior oblique view (*left*); stent is ready to be implanted (*middle*); stent is implanted in the proper place with dilatation of the stenosis (*right*)

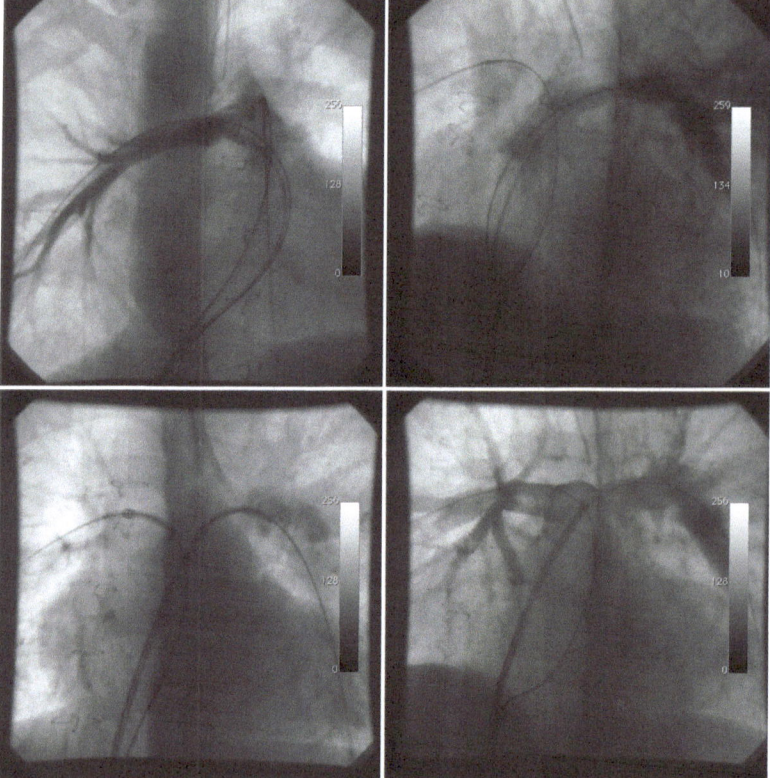

Fig. 11.3 Bilateral moderate hypoplasia of both pulmonary arteries. Right pulmonary artery angiography in right anterior oblique view (*upper left*); left pulmonary artery angiography in left anterior oblique angulation (*upper right*); fluoroscopy in cranial and left anterior oblique angulation showing two stent-balloon assembly at the origin of the two pulmonary arteries (*bottom left*); angiography showing the two stents in place with significant increase of vessel diameter (*bottom right*)

ed to the largest diameter (eventually to the normal vessel diameter). In our Center we do not use self-expanding stents because of the inability to redilate, diminished hoop strength, and some concern over possible increased neointimal buildup.

The balloon used to deliver the stent is chosen to be more or less equal in size to the normal vessel adjacent to the stenosis. Once the stent has been deployed, the balloon must be carefully removed to avoid inadvertent stent embolization.

Pulmonary artery (PA) stenting results in increased PA size, reduced pressure gradients, decreased right ventricular pressure, and improved PA blood flow [12–15]. Long-term follow-up (more than 15 years) for implanted PA stents in a cohort of patients undergoing this procedure between 1989 and 1992 was published in 2010 by Law et al. [16]; the authors described a cohort of 50 patients that had 71 stents implanted with a mean follow-up of 13.2 years. ToF were 68% of patients. The gradient dropped from 43 to 8 mmHg, and the narrowest PA size increased from 4.7 to 13.4 mm. The percent of stenosis changed from 62 to 12% (all $p < 0.001$) at final catheterization. Significant in-stent restenosis and neointimal proliferation was a rare finding. A 1 mm intimal peel was almost universally seen on follow-up catheterization. Patients experienced improvement in symptoms and baseline New York Heart Association (NYHA) classification at long-term follow-up. No surgical repair was needed in patients with ToF, confirming long-lasting favorable hemodynamic and clinical effects in these patients. Pressure gradients, PA size and right ventricular pressure remained significantly improved at follow-up.

Complications, including stent migration, hemoptysis, pulmonary edema, partial or complete jailing of a side branch, thrombosis, and even death, have been reported [16–18]; the incidence is about 12%, many of these occurred during the initial stent implantation experience, and are potentially avoidable in the current era [16]. Stents placed in the PAs fracture much less frequently than those placed in RV-PA conduits, presumably because conduits are subject to extrinsic compression against the sternum [16].

Stents are amenable to further dilation to accommodate somatic growth and redilated to treat restenosis when necessary [19, 20]. Restenosis and neointimal proliferation may occur, although the modified implantation technique may be helpful to avoid these complications [20]. Such restenosis is unpredictable and occurred in 35% of previously successfully dilated pulmonary arteries. Heavy body weight was reported as the single risk factor in restenosis [21].

Physicians and surgeons who treat patients with congenital heart disease are often faced with the problem of a difficult approach to a pulmonary branch artery stenosis either percutaneously (vein access problems, difficult access owing to anatomic location, right ventricular hypertrophy etc.) or surgically (owing to scarring and postoperative adhesions, excessive pulmonary blood flow from collaterals, and even sometimes the need to implement circulatory arrest or low-flow cardiopulmonary bypass). A hybrid approach with intraoperative PA stenting is a safe and an effective technique that can be used as an alternative with excellent results. The potential advantages are: (1) the stent can be manipulated and placed under direct vision in a precise and accurate position; (2) it is a faster and easier technique compared to patch angioplasty; and (3) the duration and complexity of the cardiac catheterization may be decreased by eliminating the need for percutaneous stenting. Intraoperative fluoroscopy can be used for more accurate placement [22].

11.3   Residual Ventricular Septal Defect

A residual interventricular shunt following repair of ToF (usually poorly toler-ated) was more frequent in the past. The most common areas of shunting after ToF repair are in the postero-inferior (related to the surgeon's tendency to use more superficial sutures in this area) and antero-superior margins of the patch (related to the infundibular resection that may leave this area with more frag-ile muscular tissue) [23–24]. These are often due to intramural defects in the right ventricle, which often only become apparent after regression of the hypertrophied ventricle in the postoperative period [25].

In addition, the presence of a large residual shunt may lead to an overesti-mation of the degree of right ventricular outflow tract residual obstruction. Residual VSDs associated with significant left-to-right shunting, symptoms or cardiomegaly should be closed. Accepted surgical criterion for reoperation is Qp/Qs greater than 1.5 [26].

Repeat surgery to correct residual shunting carries a higher surgical mor-bidity and mortality, sometimes due to multiple previous operations or in some cases a higher preoperative morbidity. It may also be more difficult to localize a residual shunt using the standard right atrial approach [27]. A transcatheter approach is a safe alternative, appreciated by patients and their parents because it has less psychological impact, the time spent in hospital is shorter, the procedure causes less pain and discomfort and there is usually no need for admission to an intensive care unit [28]. It certainly is less risky from the view of another cardio-pulmonary bypass run, infection, bleeding, atriotomy and a possible ventriculotomy. The procedure is similar to that of a simple congeni-tal VSD closure. General anesthesia and transesophageal echocardiogram (TEE) are used in all cases during the procedure. All patients receive heparin (100 IU/kg) and antibiotics. Access is obtained via the femoral artery (5–6 F) and vein (6–8 F). Standard right and left heart catheterization is performed as first step of the procedure and the residual shunt is profiled angiographically using the left anterior oblique view with cranial angulation. TEE is performed to assess the shunt size and the valvar function.

As an alternative, intracardiac echocardiography may be used to monitor the procedure. Device selection is 1–2 mm greater than the VSD size. The residual VSD is crossed retrograde from the left ventricle and an arterio-venous circuit is then created. The steps are similar to those used for closure

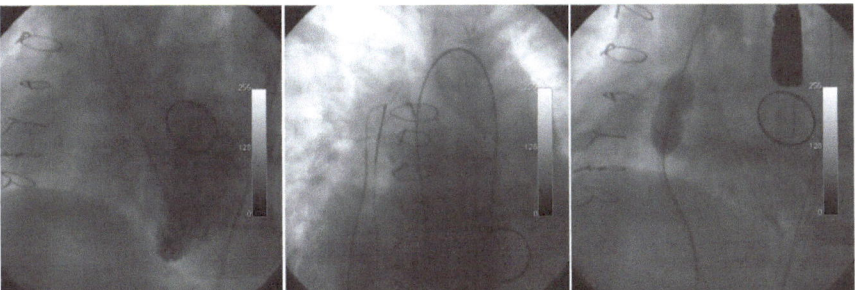

Fig. 11.4 Residual VSD in a ToF patient. Left ventricular angiography in left anterior view with cranial angulation showing a residual subaortic VSD (*left*); fluoroscopic antero-posterior view showing the creation of the artero-venous circuit (*middle*); balloon-sizing of the defect (*left*)

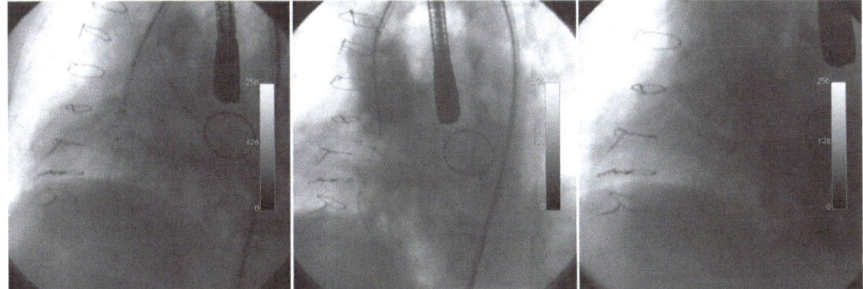

Fig. 11.5 Residual VSD in a ToF patient. Fluoroscopic view showing retrograde trans-aortic approach (*left*). The disc in the right ventricle is opened. Aortography showing no interference of the device with the aortic valve (*middle*). The device is still attached to the delivery cable; left ventricular angiography in LAO view with cranial angulation showing the device in place and no significant residual shunting (*left*)

of muscular or perimembranous defects [28–29]. In cases of residual perimembranous defects, due to the presence of the patch, it can be quite difficult to direct the tip of the long sheath towards the left ventricular apex. In these cases it is possible to leave the sheath in the ascending aorta, advance the device up to the tip of the sheath, slowly withdraw the entire unit from the aorta in the left ventricular outflow tract, and then deploy the distal disc in the left ventricle rather quickly, thus avoiding falling back into the right ventricle of the delivery system. Otherwise, a retrograde transaortic approach can be used when it is possible to use an Amplatzer muscular occlude (Figs. 11.4–11.6). In these cases, the residual defect is crossed from the left ventricle and the wire is placed in the apex of the right ventricle. The long sheath is advanced from the aorta, through the defect, and into the right ventricular apex. The device is advanced in the long sheath and then the distal disc is opened in the right ven-

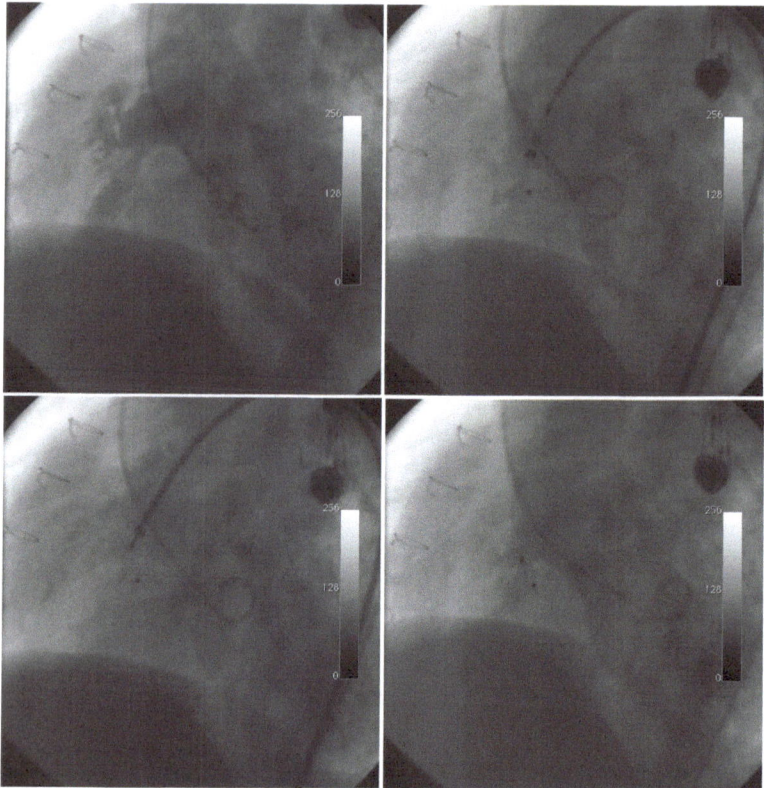

Fig. 11.6 Residual VSD in a VSD patient. Left ventricular angiography in left anterior view with cranial angulation showing a residual subaortic VSD and aneurysmal tissue around the residual defect (*upper left*); fluoroscopic view showing retrograde trans-aortic approach (*upper right*). The disc in the right ventricle is opened. Fluoroscopy showing the device deployed but still attached to the delivery cable (*bottom left*); left ventricular angiography in LAO view with cranial angulation showing the device in place and no significant residual shunting (*bottom right*)

tricle and withdrawn to the septum. The proximal disc is then opened, taking care to avoid any entrapment of the aortic valve with the disc of the device. Angiographic testing is done before releasing the device. After 10–15 minutes, the left ventricular angiogram and aortogram are repeated to assess possible residual shunting or aortic regurgitation. Throughout the procedure, the electrocardiogram is carefully screened in order to assess the occurrence of abnormalities of atrioventricular conduction or tachyarrhythmias.

Dua et al. [30] reported a series of 170 patients that underwent percutaneous VSD closure; 22 (16M) of them had residual postsurgical VSD (nine post ToF – 41%). All 22 patients had successful closure. The incidence of residual shunting was 4.5% during follow-up. One patient (post ToF correction) had a recurrent VSD due to patch dehiscence and required two transcatheter closures 2 years later; after the second recurrence she needed reoperation which was complicated by a prolonged postoperative course.

Arrhythmic problems and especially complete atrioventricular block (cAVB) are the most serious concern closing VSD, as previously reported [28–29].

In our experience only a few adult patients experienced transient arrhythmic problems (transient ventricular ectopics, acute ventricular fibrillation, atrial flutter, transient complete atrioventricular-block immediately after the implantation changed to complete right bundle branch block with sinus rhythm after 24 hours) during the procedure and these were probably related to catheter manipulation and catheter location. We did not have patients with a complete congenital atrioventricular block (cAVB) [30]. The cAVB requires pacemaker implantation, but it seems more frequent in young patients as reported by Butera et al. [29]; in that study the only variable associated with the occurrence of cAVB was age at procedure of less than 6 years. Adult patients did not experience such a complication; in 2009 we published a large series of adult patients that underwent percutaneous closure in adult age without significant arrhythmic complications [31]. Al-Kashkari et al. [32] in 2011 reported a large series where patients, despite multiple manipulations of the ventricular septum, did not experience new bundle branch blocks or other signs of intraventricular conduction delay, and also the atrioventricular (AV) node appeared to have been unaffected in all cases.

Besides, one should note that cAVB block can occur after surgical closure of a VSD in about 1% of subjects who are treated with this procedure.

The percutaneous approach showed excellent immediate and long-term results and fewer complications as compared to what has been published in the surgical approach. Percutaneous closure should therefore be the preferred method of closure for most anatomically suitable residual VSDs.

If the closure of a residual ventricular septal defect is supposed to be difficult, a transcatheter or surgically a hybrid approach may be indicated. The hybrid approach involves closing the defect through a midline sternotomy, without using cardiopulmonary bypass, by deploying a device through the right ventricle [33–34]. In any case, hybrid interventions involve close collaboration between cardiologists and surgeons and the procedures can be performed either in a theatre with fluoroscopy and transesophageal echocardiogram facilities or in a catheter laboratory with similar facilities available.

11.4   Residual Aorto-pulmonary Shunt

Transcatheter shunt closure is most often performed after definitive repair to eliminate unnecessary cardiac volume work and to decrease the risk of endocarditis. These shunts include Blalock-Taussing shunts that were not taken down at reparative surgery or that have re-canalized, and aorto-pulmonary collateral arteries that may drive excessive volume overload of the left ventricle.

Different approaches to close these shunts have been reported in recent years [35]: coil, umbrella device and plugs are the more frequent proposed devices [36–40]. The optimal technique of embolization depends on the type of the aorto-pulmonary connection, the specific anatomy and the operator preference for the device.

References

1. Chessa M, Carrozza M, Butera G et al (2006) The impact of interventional cardiology for the management of adults with congenital heart defects. Cath cardiovasc Interv 67:258-264
2. Chun Soo Park, Jeong Ryul Lee, Hong-Gook Lim et al (2010) The long-term result of total repair for TOF. Europ J Cardiothorac Surg 38:311-317
3. Hickey EJ, Veldtman G, Bradley TJ et al (2009) Late risk of outcome for adults with repaired TOF from an inception cohort spanning four decades. Eur J Cardiothorac Surg 35:156-166
4. Bacha EA, Scheule AM, Zurakowski D et al (2001) Long-term results after early primary repair of TOF. J Thorac Cardiovasc Surg 122:154-161
5. Park CS, Lee JR, Lim HG et al (2010) The long-term result of total repair for TOF. Eur J Cardiothorac Surg 38: 311-317
6. Park CS, LeeRJ, Lim HG et al (2010) The long-term result of total repair for tetralogy of Fallot. Eur J Cardiothorac Surg 38:311-317
7. Garson A Jr, Nihill MR, McNamara DG, Cooley DA (1977) Status of the adult and adolescent after repair of TOF. Circulation 59:1232-1240
8. Lock JE, Castaneda-Zuniga WR, Fuhrman BP et al (1983) Balloon dilation angioplasty of hypoplastic and stenotic pulmonary arteries. Circulation 67:962-967
9. Gentles TL, Lock JE, Perry SB et al (1993) High pressure balloon angioplasty for branch pulmonary artery stenosis: early experience. JACC 22:867-872
10. Bush DM, Hoffman TM, Del Tosario J et al (2000) Frequency of restenosis after balloon pulmonary arterioplasty and its causes. Am J Cardiol 86:1205-1209
11. Mullins C, O'Laughlin M, Vick G (1988) Implantation of balloon-expandable intravascular grafts by catheterization in pulmonary arteries and systemic veins. Circulation 77:188-199
12. Fogelman R, Nykanen D, Smallhorn JF et al (1995) Endovascular stent in the pulmonary circulation: Clinical impact on management and medium-term follow-up. Circulation 92:881-885
13. McMahon CJ, El-Said HG, Grifka RG et al (2001) Redilation of endovascular stent in congenital heart disease: Factors implicated in the development of restenosis and neointimal proliferation. J Am Coll Cardiol 38:421-426
14. O'Laughlin MP, Slack MC, Grifka RG et al (1993) Implantation and intermediate-term follow-up of stents in congenital heart disease. Circulation 88:605-614
15. Shaffer KM, Mullins CE, Grifka RG et al (1998) Intravascular stents in congenital heart disease: Short- and long-term results from a large single-center experience. J Am Coll Cardiol 31:661-666
16. Law MA, Shamszad P, Nugent AW et al (2010) Pulmonary artery stents: long-term follow-up. Catheter Cardiovasc Interv 75:757-764
17. Shaffer KM, Mullins CE, Grifka RG et al (1998) Intravascular stents in congenital heart disease: Short- and longterm results from a large single-center experience. J Am Coll Cardiol 31:661-667
18. Hwang BT, Lee PC, Fu YC et al (2000) Transcatheter stent treatment for congenital peripheral pulmonary arterial stenosis. Acta Paediatr TW 41:266-269
19. McMahon CJ, El-Said HG, Grifka RG et al (2001) Redilation of endovascular stents in congenital heart disease: Factors implicated in the development of restenosis and neointimal proliferation. J Am Coll Cardiol 38:521-526

20. Morrow WR, Palmaz JC, Tio FO et al (1993) Re-expansion of balloon-expandable stents after growth. J Am Coll Cardiol 22:2007-2013
21. O'Laughlin MP, Slack MC, Grifka RG et al (1993) Implantation and intermediate-term follow-up of stents in congenital heart disease. Circulation 88:605-614
22. Mitropoulos FA, Laks H, Kapadia N et al (2007) Intraoperative pulmonary artery stenting: an alternative technique for the management of pulmonary artery stenosis. Ann Thorac Surg 84:1338-1342
23. Pomè G, Rossi C, Colucci V et al (1992) Late reoperations after repair of TOF. Eur J Cardio Thorac Surg 6:31-35
24. Oechslin EN, Harrison DA, Harris L, Downar E (1999) Reoperation in adults with repair of TOF: indications and outcomes. J Thorac Cardiovasc Surg 118:245-251
25. Mavroudis C, Backer CL, Jacobs JP (2003) Ventricular septal defect. In: Mavroudis C, Backer CL (eds) Pediatric Cardiac Surgery, 3 edn. Philadelphia, Mosby, pp 298-320
26. Stellin G, Padalino M, Milanesi O et al (2000) Surgical closure of api- cal ventricular septal defects through a right ventricular apical intundibulatory. Ann Thorac Surg 69:597-601
27. Walsh MA, Coleman DM, Oslizlok P et al (2006) Percutaneous closure of postoperative ventricular septal defects with the Amplatzer device. Catheter Cardiovasc Interv 67:445-451
28. Carminati M, Butera G, Chessa M et al (2005) Transcatheter closure of congenital ventricular septal defect with Amplatzer septal occluders. Am J Cardiol 96:52L-58L
29. Butera G, Carminati M, Chessa M et al (2007) Transcatheter closure of perimembranous ventricular septal defects early and longterm results. J Am Coll Cardiol 50:1189-1195
30. Dua J, Carminati M, Lucente M et al (2010) Transcatheter closure of postsurgical residual ventricular septal defects: early and mid-term results. Catheter Cardiovasc Interv 75:246-255
31. Chessa M, Butera G, Negura DG et al (2009) Transcatheter closure of congenital ventricular septal defects in adult: Mid-term results and complications. Intern J of Cardiol 133:70-73
32. Al-Kashkari W, Balan P, Kavinsky CJ et al (2011) Percutaneous device closure of congenital and iatrogenic ventricular septal defects in adult patients. Catheter Cardiovasc Interv 77:260-267
33. Koch A, Bertram H, Emmel M et al (2011) Device closure of ventricular septal defects by hybrid procedures: a multicenter retrospective study. Catheter Cardiovasc Interv 77:242-251
34. Tao K, Lin K, Shi Y et al (2010) Perventricular device closure of perimembranous ventricular septal defects in 61 young children: early and midterm follow-up results. J Thorac Cardiovasc Surg 140:864-870
35. Moore JW, Ing FF, Drummond D et al (2000) Transcatheter closure of surgical shunts in patients with congenital heart disease. Am J Cardiol 85:636-640
36. Jang GY, Son CS, Lee JW (2008) Transcatheter occlusion of a modified Blalock–Taussig shunt using the Amplatzer vascular plug with the catheter–snare technique. Pediatr Cardiol 29:670-672
37. Rios-Méndez RE, Gamboa R, Mollón FP (2009) Percutaneous closure of a modified Blalock-Taussig shunt using an Amplatzer vascular plug. Rev Esp Cardiol 62:1180-1183
38. Perry SB, Radtke W, Fellows KE et al (1989) Coil embolization to occlude aortopulmonary collateral vessels and shunts in patients with congenital heart disease. J Am Coll Cardiol 13:100-108
39. Gewillig M, van der Hauwaert N, Daenen W (1990) Transcatheter occlusion of high flow Blalock-Taussig shunts with a detachable balloon. Am J Cardiol 65:1518-1519
40. Hoyer MH, Leon RA, Fricker FJ (1999) Transcatheter closure of modified Blalock-Taussig shunt with Gianturco-Grifka vascular occlusion device. Cathet Cardiovasc Interv 48:365-367

Surgical Pulmonary Valve Implantation

12

Alessandro Giamberti, Giuseppe Pomè and Alessandro Frigiola

With the increasing number of late survivors of surgeries for repair of ToF, the surgical management of the possible surgical sequelae, such as chronic pulmonary-valve insufficiency (PVI) and right ventricular (RV) dysfunction, has become a frequent problem. This is a timely topic of increasing clinical interest, as shown by the fact that pulmonary-valve replacement (PVR) for PVI is the reoperation most frequently performed today in adults with congenital heart disease (ACHD) [1, 2]. Long-standing chronic PVI, in these patients, can result in RV dilatation and failure, increasing tricuspid regurgitation, impaired exercise performance, and supraventricular or ventricular arrhythmias.

A timely reoperation of PVR may prevent these consequences, with complete RV- function recovery. The questions of when to perform a PVR, and in whom, are becoming increasingly pressing [3]. Clear guidelines to assist in this decision have proven difficult to identify. The presence of symptoms, such as from other valvular lesions, is an indubitable indication for reoperation. At our institution, all the potential candidates for PVR undergo electrocardiography, echocardiography, magnetic resonance imaging (MRI) to assess ventricular function, ventricular volume and right ventricular outflow tract (RVOT) morphology, cardiopulmonary exercise testing, and electrophysiological study.

Indications for surgery include: severe PVI (regurgitation fraction of $\geq 35\%$ on MRI); RV dilatation (RV end-diastolic volume/left ventricle [LV] end-diastolic volume ≥ 1.4 with symptoms or ≥ 2.0 without symptoms); RV systolic pressure $\geq 2/3$ of the systemic pressure with symptoms or $\geq 3/4$ without symptoms; and impaired exercise capacity (peak oxygen consumption $\leq 65\%$ of predicted value). For decision making, the following are very important: the progressive evolution of these data in the follow-up, the association with pulmonary stenosis/PVI, and the presence of peripheral pulmonary-arteries steno-

A. Giamberti (✉)
IRCCS Policlinico San Donato, Cardio-Thoracic Surgery
San Donato Milanese (Mi), Italy
e-mail: alegia@hotmail.com

M. Chessa, A. Giamberti (eds.), *The Right Ventricle in Adults with Tetralogy of Fallot,*   145
© Springer-Verlag Italia 2012

sis, severe tricuspid regurgitation, and supraventricular/ventricular arrhythmias.

The percutaneous approach now offers a less-invasive treatment that may potentially reduce the number of patients for surgery and shift the indications toward earlier intervention.

Unfortunately not all patients are good candidates for transcatheter pulmonary-valve implantation for RVOT morphology, associated cardiac anomalies, or both, and the number of surgical patients is still high.

The type of valve to be inserted into the RVOT is still debated.

Several different types of prosthesis have been used for PVR, but all are prone to failure and will likely require reintervention. At the present time, options include mechanical as well as several biological valves. Bioprosthetic valves (including homografts, xenografts, prosthetic valved conduits, and bioprosthetic valves) perform well hemodynamically, but are prone to structural degeneration that results in multiple reoperations. Mechanical valves lead to a persistent need for anticoagulation therapy, and despite some positive reports in the literature, have generally been associated with pulmonary thromboembolic complications [4, 5].

Consequently none of these valves seems to be ideal, as they all present advantages and disadvantages at the same time.

Homograft valves have been widely considered the gold standard for the reconstruction of the RVOT since their introduction into clinical practice in 1962 by Donald Ross [6]. Their results in terms of durability have been described in numerous publications [7–10], but long-term results of RVOT reconstruction with a homograft after previous correction of TOF have been scarcely reported.

In the largest published series, the authors report freedom from reoperation of 40–80% at 10 years [7–10] and the development of more than moderate homograft regurgitation at 5 years in 50–70% [11–13]. These last data become particularly relevant if the indication for repeat surgery was chronic PVI and RV failure. Homograft valves have shown the best long-term results when they are used in conjunction with pulmonary autograft replacement of the aortic valve. The results are significantly worse in non-Ross patients [13, 14]. This finding can be explained by the age of the non-Ross patients, which is usually lower than that of the Ross patients, and the normal right ventricle and normal branch pulmonary arteries of Ross patients, creating an ideal physiological environment for the implanted homograft valve.

Some authors have found homografts to be a risk factor for a second reoperation [15]. In a recent series on RVOT reconstruction for PVI after repair of ToF, of 19 patients reported, one had immediate homograft failure and has been reoperated on, three developed early PVI due to technical problems (kinking of the homograft) or rapid homograft failure [16].

This is an important topic to discuss. Homograft implantation, also for xenograft valves, and prosthetic valved conduits, requires extensive dissection of the pulmonary arteries to avoid kinking or external compression. These pulmonary-valve substitutes have a length that needs, in order to be implanted, a complete pulmonary artery dissection to avoid technical complications. Dissection can be difficult and dangerous in patients submitted to several previous surgical procedures.

A very recent study suggests that RVOT reconstruction with a homograft can be performed with low operative mortality [17]. The freedom from valve-related reoperation was 83% at 10 years and 70% at 15 years. These results are more encouraging than those reported by other investigators. Zubairi et al. [18] retrospectively analyzed the outcome of 169 consecutive patients with repaired ToF or pulmonary stenosis undergoing a first PVR using a homograft, stented porcine valve, stented porcine valve in Dacron conduit or bovine pericardial valve. The freedom from reoperation for bioprosthetic valve failure during 10 years of follow-up was excellent in all the valves used but younger age, ToF, and the use of homografts were identified as risk factors for early pulmonary valve failure.

In similar patients, Kanter et al. [19] found, at 8 years, a freedom from reoperation of 100% with porcine valves and 70% with homograft.

A more recent study by Fiore et al. [20] that directly compared three biological valves types (stented xenograft valve, bovine pericardial valve, and pulmonary homograft), concluded that the late dysfunction was more likely with homograft valves than either porcine or bovine pericardial valves. At 6 years, the freedom from explantation of the homograft was 35%.

The strategy of placing oversized homograft valves has not shown improved outcome. Karamlou and collegues [21] found that placing oversized pulmonary homograft conduits in both younger and older patients did not improve freedom from pulmonary valve failure.

All this information suggests that homografts initially have very good hemodynamic performance, but they calcify over time and become insufficient.

Finally, another problem with homograft valves is their availability. The lack of availability is difficult to quantify, but a few papers seem to show that not all the desired grafts are readily available and that availability of homograft valves is still an unsolved problem [22, 23].

Considering all these limitations, many authors now agree that homograft valves are far from ideal.

As for pulmonary-valve insertion, some surgeons now implant xenografts. Many different xenografts are available today, including porcine pulmonary-valve conduits, stentless porcine aortic-root bioprostheses, and bovine jugular valved vein conduits. The results for xenografts remain controversial at this time [8, 11, 24–27], and a longer follow-up is needed to determine the rate of structural valve deterioration and function. In any case, an extensive dissection of the pulmonary arteries, as with the homograft valves, is needed to avoid kinking due to the excessive length of the prosthesis. Extreme care must be taken during implantation, as any twisting, kinking, or external compression can easily lead to early failure [23].

The same considerations can be taken for the prosthetic valved conduits, such as Hancock or Edwards conduits.

Few papers are present in the literature regarding mechanical valves in the pulmonary position [28, 29]. Mechanical valves in the RVOT require long-term anticoagulation, subjecting the patient to the inherent risks of chronic anticoagulation therapy.

Kawachi and co-workers [30] compared St. Jude mechanical valves and bioprosthesis valves in the pulmonary position. Bioprostheses showed better performance in terms of freedom from thrombotic events, freedom from reoperation, and valve related events.

Bioprosthetic valves are probably the most widely used for pulmonary valve replacement, because they are readily available and do not need permanent anticoagulation therapy.

Shinkawa and collegues [31] analyzed the outcome and performance of bovine pericardial valves in the pulmonary position. Freedom from pulmonary valve reoperation was 100, 97.7, and 97.7% at 1, 3 and 5 years, respectively.

As previously mentioned, Kanter [19] and associates reported their experience with stented porcine valves in the pulmonary position and found that the actuarial freedom from reoperation was 100% at 8 years.

Fiore et al. [20] reported that late pulmonary valve dysfunction was lower in bovine and pericardial valves when compared with homografts.

When stratified by age, it appears that bioprostheses implanted into patients older than 10 years and with ToF have excellent durability in terms of reoperation [20].

The stentless porcine valves have been utilized extensively in the left ventricular outflow tract in adults but information on durability in the RVOT has been limited.

Hawkins and collegues [32] reported good mid-term results with the use of these valves but freedom from redo PVR for stentless porcine valves was found to be significantly lower than those for stented porcine and stented bovine pericardial valves [33].

Our approach since 2001 has been to reconstruct the RVOT with a bioprosthetic porcine valve.

Long-term durability of the bioprosthetic valves in the pulmonary position has been shown with a freedom from reoperation and freedom from complications at 10 years in more than of 85% of patients [34, 35].

We have reviewed our experience and since January 2001, 76 patients underwent RVOT reconstruction with a porcine bioprosthesis at our institution.

Severe chronic PVI was the main surgical indication in these patients. The mean age was 36 years old (with a range of 18 to 64 years old).

Sixty-five patients were ToF patients previously submitted to transannular patch repair, and 11 were patients with pulmonary stenosis (PS) previously submitted to pulmonary surgical valvulotomy. All patients had undergone previous several operations (palliative and/or corrective).

The mean time between primary cardiac repair and PVR was 28 years (with a range of 9 to 52 years).

All these patients were considered as not suitable for a percutaneous approach due to RVOT morphology, associated cardiac anomalies, or both.

Through repeated sternotomy, cardiopulmonary by-pass (CPB) was instituted in all patients. Femoral vessels were harvested in 13% of patients. No femoral cannulation was used. The mean CPB duration was 56 minutes (with a range of 44 to 101 minutes).

In 83% of our patients, the operation was performed under normothermia and under a beating heart condition. In the remaining 17%, for residual intracardiac defects requiring attention, aortic cross-clamping with cardioplegia infusion was used. In these cases, the mean aortic cross-clamping time was 30 minutes (with a range of 10 to 48 minutes).

Fifty-four patients received a bioprosthesis sized 25 mm, 14 patients received a 23 mm valve, and eight patients, a 27 mm valve.

The valves were implanted with running sutures.

Aside from the PVR, 59 patients (78%) received 95 associated cardiac surgical procedures: 33 right ventricular remodellings, 24 tricuspid-valve surgeries, 23 surgeries for arrhythmias, five residual ventricular septal defect (VSD) closures, five left pulmonary artery plasties, two residual atrial septal defect (ASD) closures, two mitral valve repairs, and one ascending aorta replacement.

The long-term outcomes of the patients were assessed through serial echocardiographic examinations and MRI control 1 year after the procedure.

There was no operative mortality.

All patients were reviewed at 6 month intervals by the referring cardiologist.

Follow-up was completed by all the patients and ranged from 6 to 132 months (mean 49 months).

Two late deaths occurred due to noncardiac problems.

All patients reported a clinical improvement and were in New York Heart Assocation (NYHA) functional class I at the last follow-up visit.

Echocardiography showed trivial or no PVI in all patients and a mean peak systolic gradient on RVOT of 19 ± 5 mm Hg.

At the 1 year MRI control, performed in 60 cases, pulmonary regurgitation fraction, right ventricular end diastolic volume (RVEDV), and RV/LV EDV improved significantly (Table 12.1).

No reoperations or valve revisions were necessary.

No episodes of structural valve deterioration, endocarditis, or thromboembolic events were noted.

Our experience is a mid-term study, and obviously, a larger follow-up is needed to determine the rate of structural valve deterioration and the function of this porcine bioprosthetic valve in the pulmonary position. These early results are encouraging, with excellent hemodynamic functioning. The bioprosthesis valves are very easy to implant and permit the avoidance of extensive

Table 12.1 Right ventricular data at 1 year magnetic resonance imaging control

Variable	Preoperative	Postoperative	P value
	Mean ±SD	Mean ± SD	
Regurgitant fraction (%)	45 ± 8	7 ± 6	0.001
RVEDV (ml/m^2)	154 ± 47	97 ± 34	0.001
RVEDV/LVEDV	2. 34 ± 0.75	1.26 ± 0.49	0.001

LVEDV, left ventricle end-diastolic volume; *RVEDV,* right ventricle end diastolic volume; *SD,* standard deviation.

dissection of the pulmonary arteries, which is particularly favorable in patients submitted multiple operations.

These excellent results with bioprosthetic valves in the RVOT may be due to the minimal hemodynamic load when placed in the pulmonary position. Orthotopic insertion of these valves with small-patch reconstruction of the RVOT permits the insertion of larger valves, reduces peel formation within the valved conduit, and eliminates external compression of the conduit [34, 35].

The bioprosthesis valves are available in all sizes and are very easy to implant. The implantation does not require dissection of the pulmonary arteries and can be performed, after a RVOT incision, with a running suture. Concerning RVOT size, the surgeon may need a small heterologous patch to close the RVOT incision on the anterior part of the valve. This small patch does not limit the possible RV-remodeling procedures that very often we must undertake during RVOT reconstruction [36].

The bioprosthetic valve does not require anticoagulation therapy and there is no risk of external compression.

Another criterion to take into consideration in the RVOT reconstruction should be the facilitation of future interventional procedures, such as percutaneous pulmonary-valve implantation. When the prosthetic valve ultimately fails, percutaneous valve implantation will reduce the number of future reoperations.

Until now, homograft valves or prosthetic valved conduits seemed to be the ideal candidates but many recent reports in the literature show the percutaneous approach is possible even in bioprosthesis valves. Percutaneous reimplantation of a pulmonary valved stent in a degenerated bioprosthetic valve has been successfully done [37, 38] and the new models of percutaneous pulmonary valves presented [39] make possible and easier the transcatheter approach in the bioprosthetic valves.

Very recently [40], a percutaneous implantation of an Edwards SAPIEN valve was successfully performed in ToF patients who had been previously operated upon and had a failing 25 mm Perimount pericardial bioprosthesis in the pulmonary position.

The size of the RVOT is critical, considering the transcatheter approach, and now thanks to the devices available, a conventional Melody valve (used in RV-PA conduits measuring less than 22 mm) or an Edwards SAPIEN valve (available in 23 or 26 mm size) can be used inside a homograft/conduit or as a "valve in valve".

In conclusion, despite the recent introduction of the transcatheter approach, the number of patients who need surgical pulmonary valve implantation is still high.

There is not an ideal valve in the pulmonary position and the choice should take into consideration the simplicity of the surgical approach and the future possibility of a percutaneous approach.

PVR using biological stented valves can be accomplished with low perioperative mortality and morbidity, and favorable mid-term clinical and excellent mid-term valve function. Longer follow-up is necessary to further evaluate the performance of this prosthesis in the pulmonary position.

References

1. Srinathan SK, Bonser RS, Sethia B et al (2004) Changing practice of cardiac surgery in adult patients with congenital heart disease. Heart 91:207-212
2. Giamberti A, Chessa M, Abella R et al (2009) Morbidity and mortality risk factors in adults with congenital heart disease undergoing cardiac reoperation. Ann Thorac Surg 88:1284-1289
3. Harrild DM, Berul CI, Cecchin F et al (2009) Pulmonary valve replacement in tetralogy of Fallot. Impact on survival and ventricular tachycardia. Circulation 119:445-451
4. Rosti L, Murzi B, Colli AM et al (1998) Mechanical valves in the pulmonary position: a reappraisal. J Thorac Cardiovas Surg 115:1074-1079
5. Waterbolk TW, Hoendermis ES, den Hamer IJ, Ebels T (2006) Pulmonary valve replacement with a mechanical prosthesis. Promising results of 28 procedures in patients with congenital heart disease. Eur J Cardiothorac Surg 30:28-32
6. Ross DN (1962) Homograft replacement of the aortic valve. Lancet 2:487
7. Boethig D, Goerler H, Westhoff-Bleck M et al (2007) Evaluation of 188 consecutive homografts implanted in pulmonary position after 20 years. Eur J Cardiothorac Surg 32:133-142
8. Boethig D, Thies WR, Hecker H, Breymann T (2005) Mid-term course after pediatric right ventricular outflow tract reconstruction: a comparison of homografts, porcine xenografts and Contegras. Eur J Cardiothorac Surg 27:58-66
9. Lange R, Weipert J, Homann M et al (2001) Performance of allografts and xenografts for right ventricular outflow tract reconstruction. Ann Thorac Surg 71:S365-367
10. Meyns B, Jashari R, Gewillig M et al (2005) Factors influencing the survival of cryopreserved homografts. The second homograft performs as well as the first. Eur J Cardiothorac Surg 28:211-216
11. Dittrich S, Alexi-Meskishvili VV, Yankah AC et al (2000) Comparison of porcine xenografts and homografts for pulmonary valve replacement in children. Ann Thorac Surg 70:717-722
12. Homann M, Haehnel JC, Mendler N et al (2000) Reconstruction of the RVOT with valved biological conduits: 25 years experience with allografts and xenografts. Eur J Cardiothorac Surg 17:624-630
13. Selamet Tierney ES, Gersony WM et al (2005) Pulmonary position cryopreserved homografts: durability in pediatric Ross and non-Ross patients. J Thorac Cardiovasc Surg 130:282-286
14. Caldarone CA, McCrindle BW, Van Arsdell GS et al (2000) Independent factors associated with longevity of prosthetic pulmonary valves and valved conduits. J Thorac Cardiovasc Surg 120:1022-1030

15. Mohammadi S, Belli E, Martinovic I et al (2005) Surgery for right ventricle to pulmonary artery conduit obstruction: risk factors for further reoperation. Eur J Cardiothorac Surg 28:217-222
16. Ghez O, Tsang VT, Frigiola A et al (2007) Right ventricular out flow reconstruction for pulmonary regurgitation after repair of tetralogy of Fallot: preliminary results. Eur J Cardiothorac Surg 31:654-658
17. Van de Woestijne PC, Mokhles MM, de Jong PL et al (2011) Right ventricular outflow tract reconstruction with an allograft conduit in patients after tetralogy of Fallot correction: long-term follow-up. Ann Thorac Surg 92:161-166
18. Zubairi R, Malik S, Jaquiss RDB et al (2011) Risk factors for prosthesis failure in pulmonary valve replacement. Ann Thorac Surg 91:561-565
19. Kanter KR, Budde JM, Parks WJ et al (2002) One hundred pulmonary valve replacements in children after relief of right ventricular outflow tract obstruction. Ann Thorac Surg 73:1801-1807
20. Fiore CA, Rodefeld M, Turrentine M et al (2008) Pulmonary valve replacement: a comparison of three biological valves. Ann Thorac Surg 85: 1712-1718
21. Karamlou T, Ungerleider RM, Alsoufi B et al (2005) Oversizeng pulmonary homograft conduits does not significantly decrease allograft failure in children. Eur J Cardiothorac Surg 27:548-553
22. Sinzobahamvya N, Wetter J, Blaschszok HC et al (2001) The fate of small-diameter homografts in the pulmonary position. Ann Thorac Surg 72:2070-2076
23. Goffin YA, Van Hoeck B, Jashari R et al (2000) Banking of cryopreserved heart valves in Europe: assessment of a 10-years operation in the European Homograft Bank (EHB). J Heart Valve Dis 9:207-214
24. Brown JW, Ruzmetov M, Rodefeld MD et al (2006) Valved bovine jugular vein conduits for right ventricular outflow reconstruction in children: an attrattive alternative to pulmonary homograft. Ann Thorac Surg 82:909-916
25. Gober V, Berdat P, Pavlovic M et al (2005) Adverse mid-term outcome following RVOT reconstruction using the Contegra valved bovine jugular vein. Ann Thorac Surg 79:626-631
26. Erez E, Tam VK, Doublin NA, Stakes J (2006) Repeat right ventricular outflow tract reconstruction using the Medtronic freestyle porcine aortic root. J Heart Valve Dis 15:92-96
27. Hartz RS, Deleon SY, Lane J et al (2003) Medtronic freestyle valves in right ventricular outflow tract reconstruction. Ann Thorac Surg 76:1896-1900
28. Rosti L, Murzi B, Colli AM et al (1998) Pulmonary valve replacement: a role for mechanical prostheses? Ann Thorac Surg 65:889-890
29. Haas F, Schreiber C, Horer J et al (2005) Is there a role for mechanical valved conduits in the pulmonary position? Ann Thorac Surg 79:1662-1667
30. Kowachi Y, Masuda M, Tominaga R et al (1991) Comparative study between St. Jude Medical and bioprosthetic valves in the right side of the heart. Jpn Circ J 55:553-562
31. Shinkawa T, Anagnostopoulos PV, Johnson NC et al (2010) Performance of bovine pericardial valves in the pulmonary position. Ann Thorac Surg 90:1295-1300
32. Hawkins JA, Sower CT, Lambert LM et al (2009) Stentless porcine valves in the right ventricular outflow tract: improved durability? Eur J Cardiothorac Surg 35:600-605
33. Lee C, Park CS, Lee CH et al (2011) Durability of bioprosthetic valves in the pulmonary position: long-term follow-up of 181 implants in patients with congenital heart disease. J Thorac Cardiovasc Surg 142:351-358
34. Yemetz IM, Williams WG, Webb GD et al (1997) Pulmonary valve replacement late after repair of tetralogy of Fallot. Ann Thorac Surg 64:526-530
35. Fukada J, Morishita K, Komatsu K et al (1997) Influence of pulmonic position on durability of bioprosthetic heart valve. Ann Thorac Surg 64:1678-1680
36. Frigiola A, Giamberti A, Chessa M et al (2006) Right ventricular restoration during pulmonary valve implantation in adults with congenital heart disease. Eur J Cardiothorac Surg 29 (Suppl I) S279-285

37. Pedra CA, Justino H, Nykanen DG et al (2002) Percutaneous stent implantation to stenotic bioprosthetic valves in the pulmonary position. J Thorac Cardiovasc Surg 124:82-87
38. Bay Y, Zong GJ, Jiang HB et al (2009) Percutaneous reimplantation of a pulmonary valved stent in sheep: a potential treatment for bioprosthetic valve degeneration. J Thorac Cardiovasc Surg 138:733-737
39. Schierano S, Coats L, Migliavacca F et al (2007) Variation in right ventricular outflow tract morphology following repair of congenital heart disease: implications for percutaneous pulmonary valve implantation. J Cardiovasc Magn Reson 9:687-695
40. MacDonald ST, Carminati M, Butera G (2011) Percutaneous implantation of an Edwards SAPIEN valve in a failing pulmonary bioprosthesis in palliated Tetralogy of Fallot. Eur Heart J [Epub ahead of print]

Other Surgical Procedures

13

Alessandro Giamberti

13.1 Introduction

ToF is the most common form of cyanotic congenital heart disease. If left untreated, it carries 33% mortality in the first year of life and 50% mortality in the first 3 years of life [1]. There are few patients with ToF that reach adulthood in natural history or after one or more palliative procedures.

Usually the majority of surgical procedures that we are performing in adult ToF patients are reoperations after total repair performed as infants or children.

We know, from the largest published series [2–4] that, for the children with ToF repaired in the modern era, the early surgical mortality is less than 2% and we can expect, for them, a 40-year survival around 90%. At the same time we know today that 30 years after correction, half of survivors needed reoperation [2–4].

With the increasing number of late survivors of surgeries for repair of ToF, the surgical management of the possible surgical sequelae, such as chronic pulmonary-valve insufficiency (PVI) and right ventricular (RV) dysfunction, has become a frequent problem.

Pulmonary-valve replacement (PVR) for PVI, represents today the most frequent reoperation performed not only in ToF patients, but in all adults with congenital heart disease (ACHD) [5, 6]. Long-standing chronic PVI can result in RV dilatation and failure, RV aneurysm, increasing tricuspid regurgitation, impaired exercise performance, and supra-ventricular or ventricular arrhythmias.

A. Giamberti (✉)
IRCCS Policlinico San Donato, Cardio-Thoracic Surgery
San Donato Milanese (Mi), Italy
e-mail: alegia@hotmail.com

Reoperation may also be required to close a residual ventricular septal defect (VSD) or to close a permeable foramen ovale or atrial septal defects (ASD) not closed at the correction that can be the cause of paradoxical embolism in some cases.

Finally, despite excellent results after Tetralogy of Fallot (ToF) repair, a cohort of patients develop progressive aortic dilatation and subsequent aortic valve incompetence, needing reoperation on the aortic root.

Not all these surgical sequelae, especially if isolated, have a clear indication to be surgically treated. Very often they represent "associated surgical procedures" usually done concomitantly with the surgical PVR.

We reviewed a series of 76 consecutive patients (Chap. 12) submitted to surgical PVR at our institution since 2001, and a very high number of patients (78%) received several associated cardiac surgical procedures. The most frequent were RV remodelling, tricuspid valve repair, and arrhythmia surgery.

RV dysfunction, dilatation and aneurysm, arrhythmias, and developing of secondary tricuspid valve regurgitation are complications related to long-standing/chronic PVI, and this suggests that we are probably operating on these patients too late [6–11].

Cardiac reoperations in these patients present major difficulties in management and technique. In the past a repeat sternotomy represented a technical challenge for the surgeon, but carried a significant risk of patient morbidity and death. Recent series [6, 7] demonstrate that if approached meticulously and in large centers, where reoperations are frequently performed, repeat sternotomy can represent a negligible risk of injury and subsequent morbidity and mortality.

ACHD are a growing and changing population [5, 6] of increasing clinical interest but few studies have been published on perioperative risk factors.

The only available data [6, 8, 9] suggest that reoperations in these patients are associated with a low mortality but severe morbidity is relatively frequent and is generally associated with some preoperative (high hematocrit due to cyanosis, presence of congestive heart failure, and number of previous operations) and operative (more complex operations and cardiopulmonary bypass duration) factors.

13.2   Tetralogy of Fallot Repair

Approximately only 2% of all the untreated patients with ToF reach the fourth decade of life [12]; however, there are still a certain number of older patients with uncorrected ToF. More recently, the number of operations for ToF has increased again due to the growing influx of patients from underdeveloped countries. Indications for corrective surgery in this specific population remain controversial, due to higher operative risks and doubtfully beneficial effects. These patients survive until adulthood because of favorable morphologic conditions such as systemic-to-pulmonary collaterals, a palliative shunt procedure performed in childhood, or because of relatively mild stenosis of the right ventricular outflow tract (RVOT).

These patients represent a high-risk population. Chronic hypoxemia stimulates the development of large systemic-to-pulmonary collaterals that increase the pulmonary blood flow, and together with myocardial hypertrophy and myocardial hypoxia, they lead to reduced biventricular function. Impaired ventricular function, severe and chronic hypoxemia with high hematocrit due to cyanosis, and tricuspid regurgitation are associated with higher operative mortality [6, 13].

The surgical mortality for these patients in the literature [13–17] is not irrelevant; ranging between 2.5 and 24%. A complete preoperative evaluation including cardiac catheterization and MRI must be performed in all patients. Systemic-to-pulmonary collaterals can be preoperatively closed in the cath lab.

A median sternotomy and standard aortic and bicaval cannulation is routinely applied. All the previous shunts or collaterals should be dissected out before heparin administration and divided or ligated just after cardiopulmonary bypass is commenced. The operation is performed on cardiopulmonary bypass with moderate hypothermia. The left side of the heart is vented through the right superior pulmonary vein or by direct suction through the foramen ovale. In patients with extensive bronchial collaterals, even lower temperature can be employed (around 20°C). Cold antegrade crystalloid cardioplegia is usually used.

The intracardiac repair includes VSD closure and RVOT obstruction relief. The VSD can be closed through the tricuspid valve or a right ventriculotomy. We use a heterologous pericardial patch with a running suture reinforced by additional stitches. Transpulmonary/transventricular approach is often used for the RVOT obstruction relief. After a complete resection of obstructing muscle bundles in the RVOT, the pulmonary valve is probed using graded dilators. If the valve is too small, through an incision in the pulmonary trunk, a full commissurotomy is performed. If the pulmonary annulus is still small (20 mm is accepted in adults patients), a transannular pericardial patch should be implanted. Related to preoperative myocardial hypertrophy, myocardial hypoxia, and impaired ventricular function, it seems possible that postoperative pulmonary regurgitation, in these selected patient populations, is not tolerated. When the valve cannot be preserved, some experienced groups [13, 15–17] suggest, for these patients, a routine PVR, since the PVI is less tolerated in adults than in children. Fortunately a transannular patch is required more often in children than in adulthood. In the adult ToF, usually the diameter of the pulmonary annulus is of adequate size, since those patients have been able to survive for decades without any intervention. The biggest series report, for a more favorable anatomy in adulthood, the need for transannular patch in 10 to 41% of patients [13, 15–17].

Severe postoperative bleeding that needs early surgical revision is frequently reported [13, 15, 16] affecting 10 to 20% of patients.

In contrast to the perioperative course, long-term survival has been reported to be excellent [13], comparable as great as 35 years after correction, with the life expectancy of the general population.

Not only the long-term survival, but also functional status has been reported to be excellent with a significant improvement in New York Heart Association (NYHA) functional class [15–17]. At follow-up, 75% of these patients have a normal life with full-time work, more than 65% are married and 70% of women had delivered children.

We strongly believe that despite the higher perioperative mortality, uncorrected adult ToF clearly benefits from total correction because the functional status improves markedly.

13.3   RV Remodeling

The physiologic consequences of chronic PVI in adult patients who underwent ToF repair include progressive RV dilatation and dysfunction, and the typical treatment has traditionally been PVR. However, correction of the inciting lesion of pulmonary insufficiency may not be sufficient treatment to allow RV recovery, when PVR is performed at either an advanced stage of RV failure and/or when it is done in the presence of the structural defect of either aneurysm or akinesia of a portion of the RVOT [10, 11, 18, 19].

The implications of these aneurysmal or akinetic lesions are that they disrupt RV structure and thereby produce functional alterations of the physiologic peristaltic RV contraction pattern that proceeds from the RV inlet towards the outlet: a contractile sequence that is heavily dependent upon RV geometric configuration.

Recognition, today, of the deleterious functional consequences of the aneurysm or akinetic lesions of RVOT suggest to the surgeon to include surgical treatment of these ventricular wall defects at the time of PVR.

Several factors account for the aneurysm or akinesia of the RVOT after repair of ToF. The anatomic contributers include prior placement of a large transannular or infundibular patch, as well as aggressive myomectomy during infundibular resection. There may also be an ischemic insult resulting from conal arterial branch interruption during suture placement area around the patch.

The surgical treatment of the aneurysm or akinesia of the RVOT, so-called RV remodeling, starts by removing the previous transannular or infundibular patch. All the aneurysmatic tissue in the RVOT is removed and the functioning edges of the adjacent RV muscle are identified. Related to the altered RV geometry, a more longitudinal [20] or circular [10] ventriculoplasty is done. We prefer the circular one [10] to reduce RV volume. A continuous 2-0 Goretex suture is placed all around the previously identified still functioning muscular edges (including the septal area) and by pulling the two ends of the suture towards the pulmonary annulus in order to create a RVOT dimension that is able to accept a 26 mm Hegar dilator to insure absence of restriction. The two ends of the Goretex suture are then fixed at the level of the pulmonary valve annulus, with the dilator in place. After removing the dilator, a pulmonary valve is implanted, and a small Dacron/pericardial patch is placed over the reduced ventriculoplasty and pulmonary arteriotomy to close these openings.

13.4   Tricuspid Valve Surgery

Tricuspid valve regurgitation (TR) is a well known possible complication in adult ToF patients after complete repair, and can be associated with different anatomical or functional mechanisms. An anatomical mechanism is when the tricuspid valve is damaged by previous operations. In some patients the septal leaflet of the tricuspid valve (TV) becomes distorted by the patch used to close the VSD or by a fibrotic reaction to this patch.

Functional TR is the consequence of right ventricular (RV) dilation or dysfunction. RV dilation/dysfunction is typically associated with chronic volume overloading related to long-standing PVI after previous repair of ToF. The physiologic consequences of chronic RV volume overloading in these patients can compromise tricuspid valve function.

In the absence of anatomical modification or damage, the TR is associated with a tricuspid annulus and hence RV dilatation.

Very often, adults with repaired ToF with chronic PVI present associated moderate to severe TR via annulus dilatation and adverse leaflet tethering due to left-sided septal bulging, a secondary consequence of the RV dilation.

The number of patients with functional TR will increase in the near future as will the incidence of ACHD. In an analysis of our activity [21], the surgical treatment of functional TR was required in 32% of our patients submitted to surgical PVR.

Moderate to severe TR is a clear indication for surgical treatment.

It was thought in the past that the severity of secondary or functional TR decreases or even disappears after correction of the primary lesion. This concept, widely supported in the past, has influenced current practice regarding conservative management of secondary TR.

As demonstrated in the functional TR secondary to mitral lesions, TR does not spontaneously disappear once the left lesion has been corrected. The data demonstrate that once the annulus is dilated and RV function is therefore mildly impaired, the process of TR is progressive and will subsequently become clinically relevant. Once the RV is dilated, it is not enough to treat the cause of the RV volume overload (PVR) alone. Such an approach does not correct TV dilation. Once the TV annulus is dilated, its size cannot spontaneously return to normal and it may continue to dilate further.

TR continues to impact right ventricular function, which may explain why some patients require a secondary operation for the TR years after the first lesion has been repaired surgically.

The hospital mortality is extremely high with regard to reoperation for isolated secondary severe TR [22] and medical treatment for these patients is rather limited and inefficient. It has therefore been recommended by some experts that a more aggressive approach should be taken in cardiac surgery patients with concomitant TR [21, 23, 24].

Obviously, tricuspid valve repair is preferable to tricuspid valve replacement. It remains unclear which techniques are optimal for repair of the tricuspid valve. Although Key's and De Vega's techniques are reproducible and have been widely used for suture annuloplasty, the residual recurrence of moderate to severe TR among hospital survivors was reported in 16–34% of cases [25, 26]. It has therefore been recommended that such patients undergo tricuspid valve repair with an annuloplasty ring [27, 28]. The ring annuloplasty remodels the annulus, decreases tension on suture lines, increase leaflets coaptation, and prevents recurrent annulus dilation.

Unfortunately, TV repair is not always possible, especially when the mechanism of TR is more anatomical than functional.

In cases of tricuspid valve replacement, bioprosthesis is preferable. Previous reports [29, 30] show that bioprostheses in the tricuspid position are more satisfactory than mechanical valves, resulting in favorable long-term outcomes, a low incidence of structural valve deterioration and reoperation.

13.5   Arrhythmias Surgery

Supraventricular and ventricular arrhythmias are an important cause of morbidity and mortality in adult patients with severe PVI who had previously undergone ToF surgical repair. The physiologic consequences of PVI include progressive right ventricular dilatation and dysfunction followed by a secondary long-standing complication like tricuspid valve dysfunction and atrial and/or ventricular arrhythmias due to atrial or ventricular stretch that require a more complex surgical approach associated with the simple pulmonary valve implantation [6, 10, 11, 21, 31].

Arrhythmias are a major cause of morbidity and mortality and one of the most important reasons for hospitalization in adults with ToF. Arrhythmias that might be considered benign in patients with a normal heart may lead to catastrophic hemodynamic deterioration and be life-threatening in patients with surgical sequelae.

Atrial and ventricular arrhythmias have been consistently reported during the follow-up of patients who have undergone repair of ToF, with sudden cardiac death being the most common cause of mortality late after the repair. The incidence of arrhythmias in these patients ranges from 2 to 23% for atrial arrhythmias and from 14 to 65% for ventricular arrhythmias [32–34]. Sustained ventricular tachycardia is present in more than 20% of these patients, with a risk of late sudden death ranging from 2 to 6% over a follow-up of 18.5 ± 9.6 years [34–36]. An important concept is that an arrhythmia presenting prior to cardiac surgery is not modified by the surgical treatment of the congenital defect alone; consequently, arrhythmia surgery should be taken into consideration for these patients. Arrhythmias will persist in a high percentage of patients following surgery unless the arrhythmia itself is specifically treated. The recent development of transcatheter ablative techniques to treat various forms of arrhythmias has largely eliminated routine surgical ablation. The surgical approach is now reserved for patients in whom transcatheter ablation procedures have failed or for patients with associated structural cardiac defects requiring concomitant surgery. Intraoperative ablation creating endocardial linear lines of conduction block offers an alternative to complex surgical techniques such as the Cox-Maze procedure.

The current approach for these patients undergoing repeat surgery is a preoperative assessment of atrial and ventricular arrhythmias including 24-hour electrocardiographic monitoring, exercise testing and electrophysiologic studies with programmed ventricular stimulation for patients with symptoms due to arrhythmia [31]. Atrial arrhythmias can be treated by a right-sided Maze procedure at the time of reoperation [31]. Sustained ventricular tachycardia may be treated at the time of reoperation with direct endocardial resection or ablation [31].

Close collaboration with the electrophysiologists is required. Except for patients with atrial fibrillation (AF), all the other candidates need preoperative electrophysiologic studies in order to identify the different electyrophysiologic substrates and mechanisms of arrhythmia.

The surgical treatment of arrhythmias is not an alternative but rather an eventual adjunct to catheter ablation procedures. Arrhythmia surgery is reserved for patients in whom the catheter ablation technique fails and the procedures can be easily and successfully incorporated into the surgical treatment.

Since the 1980s, the Cox-Maze III operation has been the surgical procedure of choice for the management of medically refractory AF. Nevertheless, the Cox-Maze III operation remains a complex procedure requiring lengthy surgery and prolonged cardiopulmonary bypass; furthermore, it is associated with a high incidence of bleeding requiring reopening of the chest, and with the risk of late pulmonary vein stenosis.

Many modifications have been developed recently in an attempt to simplify the technique. These include changes in atriotomies and the replacement of the multiple surgical incisions by linear lesions created by alternative energy sources such as cryoablation, dry radiofrequency ablation or irrigated radiofrequency ablation.

The problem of these ablation techniques in the presence of a congenital heart defect is the thickness of the atria and the variance of the anatomy. The objective of intraoperative ablation is to obtain a reliable transmural line of block despite the thick atria.

We use the irrigated monopolar radiofrequency technique. As previously reported, [31, 37, 38] there have been no unforeseen complications resulting from the use of irrigated radiofrequency and based on our experience, we can confirm that this is a simple to use and effective system.

Our current policy is to perform Cox Maze III ablation in the presence of preoperative AF and to reserve the use of the modified right-sided Maze ablation for patients with preoperative episodes of atrial flutter and/or supraventricular tachycardia. Ablation lines and surgical incisions are performed in a standard way in the right and left atria and have been previously reported [37]. Sustained ventricular tachycardia may be treated at the time of reoperation by direct endocardial resection, cryoablation or radiofrequency ablation. Postoperative (6 months later) programmed ventricular stimulation is necessary to determine the efficacy of the treatment and, if sustained tachycardia remains inducible, a defibrillator should be implanted.

13.6 Residual VSD/ASD

Reoperation for residual VSD after ToF repair was quite frequent in the past [39] but fortunately the incidence has recently decreased.

In general, reoperation is advised for isolated residual VSD when the Qp/Qs is 1.5 or greater. Rarely is such a big residual VSD, after ToF repair, tolerated until adulthood; the majority are small residual VSD that are closed concomitant with other surgical procedures, especially PVR.

The commonest location is in the posteroinferior quadrant near the area of the conduction tissue. This may be related to the surgeon's tendency to use more superficial sutures in this area. The second typical location is the anterosuperior quadrant, which may be related to the infundibular resection that may leave this area with more fragile muscular tissue.

Related to the size of the defect, one can use a second patch or direct closure with pledgeted sutures.

Especially for the anterosuperior location, very often the tissue around the defect is completely calcified, making it difficult to pass stitches. The problem can be easily solved with a hybrid approach using a transcatheter VSD device during the operation.

Similarly, a reoperation for isolated ASD is advised when a significant (Qp/Qs greater than 1.5) residual shunt is present.

The presence of a simple patent foramen ovale (PFO) must be accurately detected before any possible reoperation in adult ToF to avoid risks of air embolism during surgery.

13.7 Dilated Ascending Aorta, Aortic Regurgitation

In 1997 the first series on progressive aortic root dilatation in repaired ToF was published by the Mayo Clinic group [40]. The report mentioned that, despite excellent results after ToF repair, a substantial cohort of patients developed progressive aortic dilatation and subsequent aortic valve incompetence, needing reoperation on the aortic root.

It is common for the ascending aorta and aortic root in conotruncal anomalies like ToF to be dilated at birth and at initial repair.

The pathophysiology of aortic root dilatation in these patients is a combination of increased aortic blood flow before complete repair, and intrinsic vascular structural anomalies.

Niwa and collegues [41] examined aortic specimens from patients with congenital heart defects and all the aortic specimens of the conotruncal defects had medial wall abnormalities of smooth muscle, elastic fibers, collagen, and ground substance.

At the same time, progressive aortic root dilatation has been reported in relation to patient factors such as right aortic arch, male sex, palliative shunt before repair, and late repair [42, 43].

A recent series [44] from the Mayo Clinic group analyzed the reoperations performed on the aortic root, ascending aorta, or aortic valve in adult patients with conotruncal anomalies over a long period (1973–2008). This paper shows interesting results.

The incidence is low, and the early mortality for these operations is very low. The majority of reoperations were required for aortic valve dysfunction and not for ascending aorta dilatation. The presence of ascending aorta dilatation is usually not the main indication for operation. The indications and timing for reoperation, in these patients, more often revolves around the pathology of the RVOT, especially PVI [44]. Most of these patients come to medical attention because of right-sided problems and the aorta is accidentally found to be dilated.

The risk of ascending aorta dissection or progressive aortic dilatation requiring intervention is very low [44].

Despite enthusiasm for prophylactic operations on the ascending aorta in patients with acquired heart disease or bicuspid aortic valve disease, the moderately dilated aorta in adult ToF may be managed by observation alone. Potential important explanations for the rare occurrence of aortic dissection in these patients include the low incidence of hypertension and smoking in adults with congenital heart disease. Current consensus recommendations for adult patients with congenital heart disease are to repair ascending aorta when it is 55 mm or larger. Other indications are rapid increase of size of the ascending aorta (more than 1 cm in a year), a family history of aortic dissection, and concomitant presence of moderate or worse aortic regurgitation.

If the aortic valve requires replacement, we generally prefer mechanical prosthesis, but the majority of these patients who undergo operation require PVR in addition to a procedure on the aorta or aortic valve. In these patients we suggest biological prosthesis in the pulmonary position (Chap. 12) and a mechanical valve on the left side.

References

1. Bertranou EG, Blackstone EH, Hazelrig JB et al (1978) Life expectancy without surgery in tetralogy of Fallot. Am J Cardiol 42:458-466
2. Hickey EJ, Veldtman G, Bradley TJ et al (2009) Late risk of outcome for adults with repaired tetralogy of Fallot from an inception cohort spanning four decades. Eur J Cardiothorac Surg 35:156-166
3. Bacha EA, Scheule AM, Zurakowski D et al (2001) Long-term results after early primary repair of tetralogy of Fallot. J Thorac Cardiovasc Surg 122:154-161
4. Park CS, Lee JR, Lim HG et al (2010) The long-term result of total repair for tetralogy of Fallot. Eur J Cardiothorac Surg 38:311-317
5. Srinathan SK, Bonser RS, Sethia B et al (2004) Changing practice of cardiac surgery in adult patients with congenital heart disease. Heart 91:207-212
6. Giamberti A, Chessa M, Abella R et al (2009) Morbidity and mortality risk factors in adults with congenital heart disease undergoing cardiac reoperation. Ann Thorac Surg 88:1284-1289
7. Morales DLS, Zafar F, Arrington KA et al (2008) Repeat sternotomy in congenital heart surgery: no longer a risk factor. Ann Thorac Surg 86:897-902
8. Vida VL, Berggren H, Brawn WJ et al (2007) Risk of surgery for congenital heart disease in adult: a multicentered European study. Ann Thorac Surg 83: 161-168
9. Padalino MA, Speggiorin S, Rizzoli G et al (2007) Midterm results of surgical intervention for congenital heart disease in adults: an Italian multi center study. J Thorac Cardiovasc Surg 134:106-113
10. Frigiola A, Giamberti A, Chessa M et al (2006) Right ventricular restoration during pulmonary valve implantation in adults with congenital heart disease. Eur J Cardiothorac Surg 29(Suppl I):S279-285
11. Therrien J, Siu SC, McLaughlin PR et al (2000) Pulmonary valve replacement in adults late after repair of tetralogy of Fallot: are we operating too late? J Am Coll Cardiol 36:1670-1675
12. Kirklin JW, Barrat-Boyes BG (1993) Cardiac surgery: morphology, diagnostic criteria, natural history, techniques, results, and indications, 2 edn. Churchill Livingstone, New York
13. Dittrich S, Vogel M, Dahnert I et al (1999) Surgical repair of tetralogy of Fallot in adults today. Clin Cardiol 22:460-464
14. Presbitero P, Prever SB, Contraffatto I, Morea M (1996) As originally published in 1988: Results of total correction of tetralogy of Fallot performer in adults (Updated in 1996). Ann Thorac Surg 61:1870-1873
15. Atik FA, Atik E, da Cunha CR et al (2004) Long-term results of correction of tetralogy of Fallot in adulthood. Eur J Cardiothorac Surg 25:250-255
16. Horer J, Friebe J, Schreiber C et al (2005) Correction of tetralogy of Fallot and pulmonary atresia with ventricular septal defect in adults. Ann Thorac Surg 80:2285-2292
17. Nollert GD, Fischlein T, Bouterwek S et al (1997) Long-term results of total repair of tetralogy of Fallot in adulthood: 35 years follow-up in 104 patients corrected at the age of 18 or older. Thorac Cardiovasc Surg 45:178-181
18. D'Udekem Y, Pasquet A, Van Caenegem O et al (2004) Reoperation for severe right ventricular dilatation after tetralogy of Fallot repair: pulmonary infundibuloplasty should be added to homograft implantation. J Heart Valve Dis 13:307-312
19. D'Udekem Y, Rubay J, Ovaert C (2001) Failure of right ventricular recovery of fallot patients after pulmonary valve replacement: delay of reoperation or surgical technique? J Am Coll Cardiol 37:2008-2009
20. del Nido PJ (2006) Surgical management of right ventricular dysfunction late after repair of tetralogy of Fallot: right ventricular remodeling surgery. Semin Thorac Surg Pediatr Card Surg Ann 9:29-34
21. Giamberti A, Chessa M, Ballotta A et al (2011) Functional tricuspid valve regurgitation in adults with congenital heart disease: an emerging problem. J Heart Valve Dis 20:565-570
22. Sugimoto T, Okada M, Ozaki N et al (1999) Long term evaluation of treatment for function-

al tricuspid regurgitation with regurgitant volume: characteristic differences based on primary cardiac lesions. J Thorac Cardiovasc Surg 117: 463-471

23. Cohn LH (1994) Tricuspid regurgitation secondary to mitral valve disease: when and how to repair. J Card Surg 9:237-41
24. Duran CH, Pomar JL, Colman T et al (1980) Is tricuspid valve repair necessary? J Thorac Cardiovasc Surg 80:849-860
25. Holper K, Haehnel JC, Augustin N, Schening F (1993) Surgical for tricuspid insufficiency: long term follow-up after De Vega annuloplasty. Thorac Cardiovasc Surgeon 41:1-8
26. De Paolis R, Bobbio M, Ottimo G et al (1990) De Vega tricuspid annuloplasty. Perioperative mortality and long term follow-up. J Cardiovasc Surg 31:512-517
27. Tang GH, David TE, Sing SK et al (2006) Tricuspid valve repair with an annuloplasty ring results in improved long-term outcomes. Circulation 114 (Suppl I):I-577-I-581
28. McCarthy PM, Bhudia SK, Rajeswaran J et al (2004) Tricuspid valve repair: durability and risk factors for failure. J Thorac Cardiovasc Surg 127:674-685
29. Nakano K, Eishi K, Kosakai Y et al (1996) Ten-year experience with the Carpentier-Edwards pericardial xenograft in the tricuspid position. J Thorac Cardiovasc Surg 111:605-612
30. Omata T, Kigawa I, Tohda E, Wanibuchi Y (2001) Comparison of durability of bioprostheses in tricuspid and mitral position. Ann Thorac Surg 71:S240-243
31. Giamberti A, Chessa M, Abella R et al (2008) Surgical treatment of arrhythmias in adults with congenital heart defects. Int J Cardiol 129:37-41
32. Roos-Hesselink J, Pelroth MG, McGhie J, Spitaels S (1995) Atrial arrhythmias in adults after repair of tetralogy of Fallot: correlation with clinical, exercise and echocardiographic findings. Circulation 91:2214-2219
33. Deanfield JE, McKenna WJ, Presbitero P et al (1984) Ventricular arrhythmia in repaired and unrepaired tetralogy of Fallot: relation to age, timing of repair and hemodynamic status. Br Heart J 52:77-81
34. Nollert G, Fischlein T, Bouterwek S et al (1997) Long-term survival in patients with repair of tetralogy of Fallot: 36-year follow-up of 490 survivors of the first year after surgical repair. J Am Coll Cardiol 30:1374-1383
35. Khairy P, Landzberg MJ, Gatzoulis MA et al (2004) Value of programmed ventricular stimulation after tetralogy of Fallot repair. A multicenter study. Circulation 109:1994-2000
36. Gatzoulis MA, Balaji S, Webber SA et al (2000) Risk factors for arrhythmia and sudden cardiac death late after repair of tetralogy of Fallot: a multicentre study. Lancet 365:975-981
37. Giamberti A, Chessa M, Foresti S et al (2006) Combined atrial septal defect surgical closure and irrigated radiofrequency ablation in adult patients. Ann Thorac Surg 82:1327-1331
38. Nakagawa H, Yamanashi WS, Pitha JV et al (1995) Comparison of in vivo temperature profile and lesion geometry for radiofrequency ablation with a saline-irrigated electrode versus temperature control in a canine thigh muscle preparation. Circulation 91:2264-2273
39. Pomè G, Rossi C, Colucci V et al (1992) Late reoperations after repair of tetralogy of Fallot. Eur J Cardio Thorac Surg 6:31-35
40. Dodds III GA, Warnes CA, Danielson G (1997) Aortic valve replacement after repair of pulmonary atresia and ventricular septal defect or tetralogy of Fallot. J Thorac Cardiovasc Surg 113:736-741
41. Niwa K, Perloff JK, Bhuta SM et al (2001) Structural abnormalities of great arterial walls in congenital heart disease: light and electron microscopic analyses. Circulation 103:393-400
42. Niwa K, Siu SC, Webb GD, Gatzoulis MA (2002) Progressive aortic root dilatation in adults late after repair of tetralogy of Fallot. Circulation 106:1374-1378
43. Francois K, Zaqout M, Bové T et al (2010) The fate of the aortic root after early repair of tetralogy of Fallot. Eur J Cardiothorac Surg 37:1254-1258
44. Stulak JM, Dearani JA, Burkhart HM et al (2010) Does the dilated ascending aorta in an adult with congenital heart disease require intervention? J Thorac Cardiovasc Surg 140:S52-57

Late Arrhythmias: Current Approaches

14

Sara Foresti, Maria Cristina Tavera, Pierpaolo Lupo
and Riccardo Cappato

> *"Late onset arrhythmias in adulthood appear*
> *to have become the price to pay for decades*
> *of effective hemodynamic palliation"*
> E.P.Walsh [1]

14.1 Introduction

ToF represents a good example of the many challenges in treating patients with adult congenital heart disease (ACHD). This abnormality is not infrequent, being the most common form of cyanotic congenital heart disease (CHD) after 1 year of age with an incidence of about 10% of all CHD [2]. Surgery for correction of the anatomic and hemodynamic imbalance associated with ToF was first introduced in the mid fifties and became common practice in the sixties. Continuous improvements in surgical therapy have led to a relatively large population of adult patients with ToF reaching the age of 40 to 50 years in good clinical condition and with an extended life expectancy. Despite these improvements, a significant proportion of ToF patients still present with a higher morbidity and mortality compared to the general population [3].

In various single and multicenter studies, late morbidity and mortality after repair of ToF have been reported to be caused by cardiac ventricular arrhythmias [4–6]. In a recent study by the Alliance for Adult Research in Congenital Cardiology (AARCC) in 556 patients followed until late after repair of ToF, 43.3% of the patients presented at least one episode of sustained arrhythmia or underwent electrophysiological evaluation and/or *implantable cardioverter-defibrillator* (ICD) implantation [7]. Atrial arrhythmias had a prevalence of 20.1%: in 11.5% of patients this was due to a right atrial macroreentrant tachycardia. Atrial fibrillation was more frequently (7.4%) observed in patients with older age, often in association with left side heart disease. The single most common arrhythmia was sustained ventricular tachycardia (VT), which was reported in 14.2% of the patients (Fig. 14.1).

S. Foresti (✉)
IRCCS Policlinico San Donato, Arrhythmia and Electrophysiology Center
San Donato Milanese (Mi), Italy
e-mail: sara.foresti@grupposandonato.it

M. Chessa, A. Giamberti (eds.), *The Right Ventricle in Adults with Tetralogy of Fallot*,
© Springer-Verlag Italia 2012

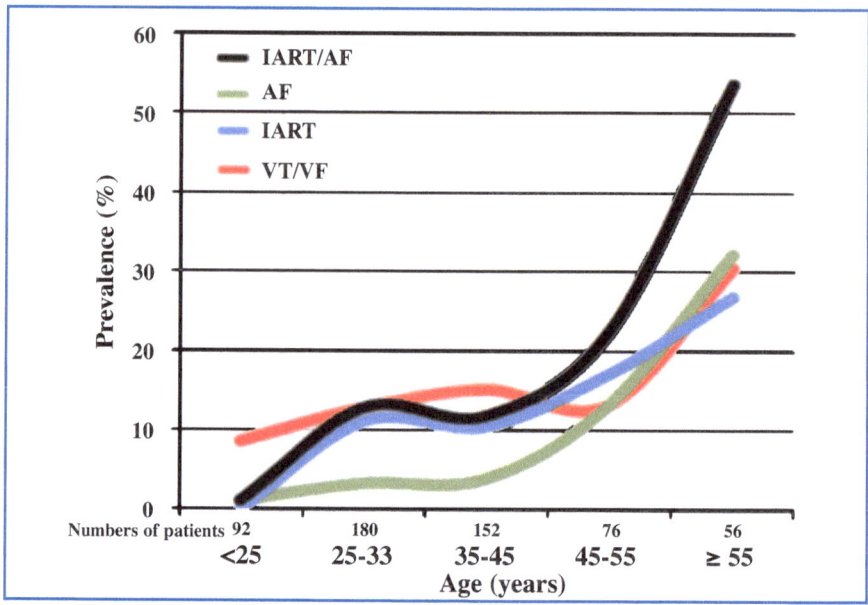

Fig. 14.1 Atrial and ventricular arrhythmia prevalence in adult patients late after repair of ToF according to age. Arrhythmic burden increases with age; ventricular and atrial tachycardia were the most common arrhythmias in younger adults, while atrial fibrillation seems to appear later (from Khairy et al. [7] with permission)

In this Chapter we will focus on sudden cardiac death and ventricular arrhythmias associated with ToF.

14.2   Correlation of Natural and Surgical Anatomy with Ventricular Arrhythmias

Precise knowledge of the underlying anatomy and the changes produced by surgical correction represents a prerequisite for a successful electrophysiological investigation in patients with CHD. The risk of developing arrhythmias after repair of ToF is influenced by the surgical approach and by the age at time of corrective surgery. In the early period, surgery was usually delayed until after the age of 5–6 years and sometimes as late as the second decade of life. This strategy usually exposed patients to longstanding pressure overload, right ventricular hypertrophy and stress from cyanosis. When corrective intervention was performed late in life many patients also received palliation surgery. In this population, volume overload further contributed to the cardiovascular distress caused by the hemodynamic condition. In the seventies, patients were proposed surgical correction at an early age due to improvement in myocardial protection and surgical techniques. This technique led to the need for a wide infundibulum resection and the use of large patches either limited to the outflow tract or extended above the pulmonary valve (trans-annular patches). The subsequent knowledge of the adverse hemodynamic effect of residual pulmonary valve regurgitation led to a further evolution of the surgical technique. At present, surgical correction is performed at an early age (~ 1 year) with the aim of preserving pulmonary valve function and avoiding wide infundibular resection and deployment of large patches. Knowledge of complete anatomical and surgical details in the single patient is also useful to assess risk stratification and arrhythmia treatment late after ToF repair.

14.3   Sudden Death

Sudden death represents one of the most frequent causes of mortality in patients with ToF. The long-term prevalence of sudden death has been reported to be 3.98% [3] reaching 8.3% at 35 years of follow-up [4] with an annual incidence of 0.15% [8] rising to 0.62% 25 years after surgery [5]. In the early days, sudden death was thought to be related to bradyarrhythmia, because of the close anatomical relationship between the ventricular septal defect (VSD) and the conduction system. Indeed, the incidence of early post-surgical *atrioventricular (*AV) block is as low as 1% whereas the occurrence of late conduction defects is very low and usually expressed by the combination of long PQ interval associated with bifascicular block [9]. The clinical characteristics of patients presenting with ventricular arrhythmias are very similar to those of patients with sudden death. This observation, together with the information obtained from ToF patients implanted with ICDs, led to the widely accepted speculation that most sudden deaths are related to ventricular arrhythmias.

14.4   Ventricular Arrhythmias

Premature ventricular contractions (PVCs) are present in 48% of patients with ToF; when Holter monitoring is available, PVC prevalence rises to 70% while sustained VT can be induced at electrophysiological study (EPS) in 9% of patients [10]. In a recent multicenter study, clinical sustained VT could be documented in 14.2% of patients [7]. First detection of PVCs can be early after surgery (2 months), but more commonly it occurs later on (up to 21 years); in more than 80% of patients, PVCs are recorded after the first postoperative year and in more than 30% PVCs still appear 10 years after surgery [11]. The occurrence of ventricular arrhythmias has been related to older age at correction, time from surgery, pulmonary valve regurgitation and high right ventricular systolic and diastolic pressure [10–12].

14.5 Mechanism of Ventricular Arrhythmias

Identification of the mechanisms underlying ventricular arrhythmias after ToF repair has long been a matter of discussion among investigators. In the early days, studies from experimental and animal models suggested a focal origin of the arrhythmias due to triggered activity. Although this is possible for PVCs, recent experience from surgical and transcatheter mapping of VT provided evidence for a re-entrant circuit as the most common mechanism of these arrhythmias. In order for re-entry to occur, the following three conditions are required: (1) two pathways with different conduction velocity; (2) differential refractoriness between the two pathways; and (3) a slowing of conduction. Comprehensibly, hemodynamic defects and surgical correction of ToF can provide a variable combination of the conditions for the re-entrant arrhythmias mentioned above. In particular, surgical incisions and prosthetic patches create the substrate for lines of block in the right ventricle facilitating re-entry. Furthermore, the overstressed and cyanotic muscular tissue in the outflow tract facilitates aneurysm formation with fibrosis and cellular disarray thus favoring conduction slowing. During electroanatomical mapping of the right ventricle (RV) recording of low amplitude, fragmented potentials is the expression of the conduction slowing that occurs in some areas of the right outflow tract. In these circumstances, the ability to pace the ventricle during VT and entrain the arrhythmia provides further confirmation of the re-entrant circuit, perpetuating the clinical arrhythmias (Figs. 14.2, 14.3).

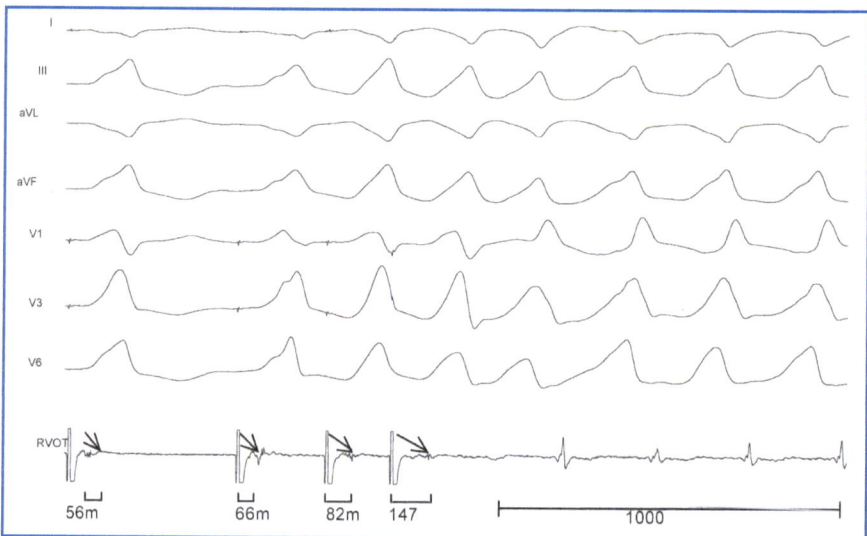

Fig. 14.2 During ventricular stimulation from RVOT pacing CL 500 ms there is a delay of > 50 ms from the stimulus to local activation suggesting delayed conduction. With extrastimulus local conduction delays with decremental proprieties facilitating reentry

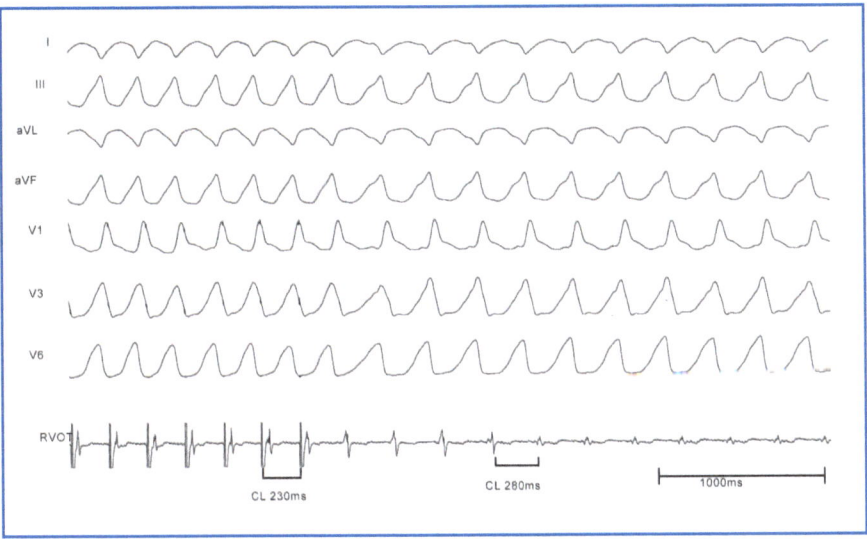

Fig. 14.3 Ineffective attempt to terminate VT by burst pacing from RVOT shows tachycardia capture with concealed fusion

14.6 The Challenge of Risk Stratification: Shooting a Moving Target

The occurrence of sudden death represents a clinically relevant problem in adult patients with repaired ToF, its incidence being not trivial and its prevalence growing rapidly. Although their risk of dying suddenly tends to grow late after surgery (i.e., decades), patients with ToF are still exposed to this risk at a mean age (i.e., 30–40 years) markedly lower than in the general population. Unfortunately, patients with ToF represent a very limited population and their relatively low incidence of sudden death prevents accurate identification of stratifiers at any time throughout their life span. In addition, the change in the timing and technique for correction has been dramatic over the years, leading to a very inhomogeneous population. As a consequence, the information collected from the early generation of adult patients with repaired ToF should be applied with caution to the next generations of ToF patients undergoing different surgical strategies.

Previous studies have shown that sudden death is more likely to occur in patients receiving surgical correction at an older age, or in patients receiving multiple interventions [3–5]. Also, it has been proven that the risk of sudden death increases as time from surgery increases and is larger if a trans-annular patch was needed [3–5, 11]. These clinical characteristics are not very helpful in stratifying the risk in older ToF patients because their prevalence in the overall ToF population is pretty large. Further evaluation to more accurately select patients who might benefit from arrhythmia prevention has been attempted by investigating a number of variables.

14.6.1 QRS Duration

A correlation between sudden death and QRS prolongation (> 180 msec) has been documented in different studies [4, 13, 14]. This is not surprising, because QRS prolongation is the electrical expression of an unfavorable evolution of the right ventricle mainly due to volume overload leading to dilatation and fibrosis (mechano-electrical interaction). QRS prolongation is a sensitive marker of an increased risk of arrhythmia, but its specificity is questionable.

14.6.2 PVC and Non-sustained VT

Recording of PVCs on Holter monitoring is a very frequent finding in ToF patients. With the exception of one study [15], high grade ectopy and non sustained VT have been associated with an higher incidence of sudden death [10, 11, 14, 16, 17].

14.6.3 Left Ventricular End Diastolic Pressure (LVEDP)

As the population of patients after repair of ToF in whom an internal ICD was implanted increases, we can learn from the device follow-up of these patients. In a recent study [17], the strongest predictor of appropriate therapy in patients with ICD implanted for primary prevention after ToF repair was an elevated left ventricular and diastolic pressure. The authors suggest that left ventricular diastolic dysfunction can be an early marker of systolic dysfunction and that its hemodynamic effects can contribute to the negative evolution of the right ventricle in the presence of a significant pulmonary valve regurgitation and volume overload [7].

14.6.4 Electrophysiological Study (EPS)

The understanding of mechanisms underlying ventricular arrhythmias after ToF repair led to the natural conclusion of trying to investigate such mechanisms during programmed electrical stimulation (PES). Early experience with PES in ToF for risk stratification was rather disappointing, but this was probably due to the very conservative protocol used (i.e., two extrastimuli) [10].

Aggressive PES (three extrastimuli with minimum coupling interval of 180 ms) was demonstrated to be effective in predicting major events, but it was limited by a high incidence of false negative tests in a population of adult patients with CHD [18]. In a more recent multicenter study, inducibility of monomorphic and polymorphic VT was a powerful predictor of future events with a sensitivity of 77.4% and a specificity of 79.5%; the predictive value of the test was larger in a subgroup of patients with clinical parameters indicative of a larger risk compared to the one of patients in whom PES was performed as a routine screening test [14].

At present, it appears unlikely single risk predictors may be identified to select ToF patients who might most benefit from an ICD implant. In fact, selection of just one predictor may be misleading in these patients. When evaluating a ToF patient we have to define the profile of that single patient, taking into account symptoms, surgical history, anatomical and hemodynamic status. PES can help identify patients more susceptible to ventricular arrhythmia in the high risk population. Young patients not presenting conventional risk factors and still experiencing spontaneous arrhythmias and unfavorable hemodynamic evolution should be followed very carefully.

14.7 Arrhythmia Management

It is a general rule when dealing with patients with ACHD and cardiac arrhythmias to first exclude a hemodynamic correctable cause of the index arrhythymia. If this turns out to be the case, then the first therapeutic measure has to be the correction, whenever possible, of the hemodynamic cause either by surgery or a percutaneous approach. Unfortunately the correction of the hemodynamic defect is sometimes not possible and often it is not sufficient to prevent arrhythmic complications.

14.7.1 Anti-arrhythmic Drug Therapy

Use of anti-arrhythmic drugs in patients with CHD is limited. Typically, class IC drugs are not administered because of their negative inotropic and proarrhythmic effect. Amiodarone is less proarrhythmic and has a less negative inotropic effect, but its long-term toxicity limits its use in patients with a long life expectancy. Beta-blockers and Sotalol are often used to control arrhythmias in patients experiencing multiple ICD shocks or presenting symptomatic PVCs. The role of Dronedarone, a newly introduced class III anti-arrhythmic drug, in adults with CHD is still to be fully evaluated, but recent evidence of significant hepatic toxicity makes its use less appealing for patients with a risk of hepatic dysfunction due to right ventricular failure.

14.7.2 Implantable Cardioverter Defibrillators (ICDs)

ICDs represent a powerful tool for the termination of ventricular arrhythmias and prevention of sudden death. They have proven effective in adult patients with CHD including ToF [17, 19]. Nevertheless, device implant is related to higher incidence of early and late complications in these patients. Lead failure is reported in up to 23% of pediatric patients with ICDs [20] and inappropriate shocks are described in 25% patients after ToF repair [17]. The incidence of device complication can be due to unfavorable vascular access and cardiac abnormality. Furthermore this young population with active lives is more exposed to develop complications. QRS prolongation and the frequent occurrence of supraventricular arrhythmia increases the risk of inappropriate shock in ICD recipients.

ICD therapy is indicated for secondary prevention in patients surviving a cardiac arrest or presenting sustained ventricular arrhythmia [2]. Given the high incidence of ICD-related complications, careful patient selection is required to identify patients who might benefit from an ICD in primary prevention using the clinical and instrumental predictors presented above. The risk of limited vascular access and the possible presence of intracardiac shunts represent a limiting factor for chronic placement of an endocardial lead.

When selected, ICD therapy for primary prevention is associated with a 7.7% yearly rate of appropriate therapy delivery [17]. This population may benefit from the recent availability of fully subcutaneous ICD systems [21].

14.7.3 Transcatheter Ablation

Radiofrequency ablation of ventricular tachycardia (VT) was first reported in the nineties [22–24] with controversial results. Advances in mapping technology, improvement of radiofrequency delivering catheters and understanding of natural and post-surgical anatomy of ToF patients has led to improvement in VT ablation results. The experience published by Zeppenfeld and co-authors [25] presents 10 years' experience with 11 patients in whom EPS and transcatheter ablation was performed for recurrent VT late after repair of right ventricular CHD (mainly ToF). In their paper, the authors reported a very interesting correlation between electrophysiological mapping and post surgical anatomy. In all patients, slowing of conduction in critical isthmuses for VT was identified in the RV outflow tract in four different areas as shown in Fig. 14.4.

After the identification of critical isthmuses, radiofrequency lesions were applied at these sites with an irrigated tip catheter to obtain conduction block resulting in non inducibility of VT. At follow-up 3/11 patients underwent control EPS and in one of them VT was still inducible. In five patients, antiarrhythmic drugs were administered after the procedure. Five of the 11 patients had an ICD implanted before or after the ablation. At a clinical follow-up of 30 months no clinical VT or sudden deaths were reported.

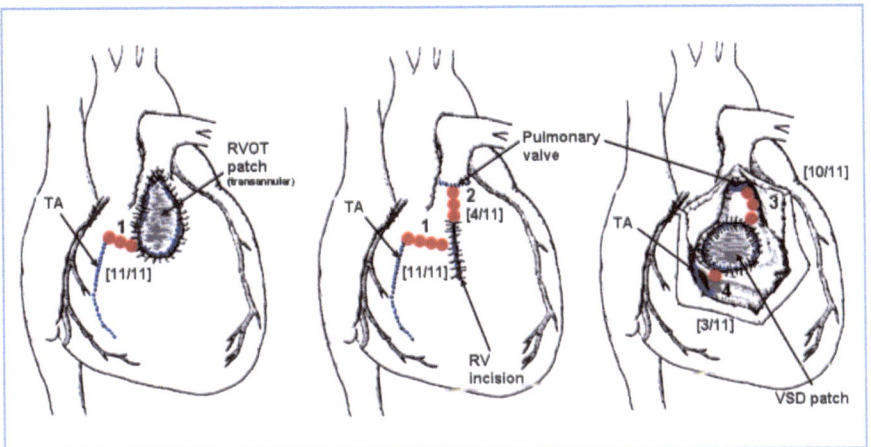

Fig. 14.4 Schematic representation of anatomic boundaries and surgical line of block (ventriculotomy) in repaired ToF and resulting anatomic isthmuses favouring VT re-entry (from Zeppenfeld et al. [25], with permission)

Results from transcatheter ablation of VT after repair of ToF are promising, but evidence of long-term efficacy in a large cohort is still lacking. Since VT has been correlated with the risk of sudden death in this population, at this time, we think that the patients presenting with clinical sustained ventricular arrhythmias should be protected with an ICD. Transcatheter ablation should be performed in association or as an alternative to anti-arrhythmic drug therapy in patients experiencing device appropriate therapies.

14.8 Role of Cardiac Surgery in Ventricular Arrhythmia

The role of a careful clinical and hemodynamic evaluation of patients with CHD experiencing arrhythmias has already been outlined in the previous sections. Surgical or percutaneous correction of significant cardiac defects represents the first line treatment to optimally approach any arrhythmogenic substrate. The single most common cause of re-intervention after ToF repair is represented by pulmonary valve regurgitation that can be corrected either by surgical or transcatheter valve placement. The controversial topic of indication and timing for intervention on the pulmonary valve is discussed in others chapters of this book. We intend to focus our attention on the impact of pulmonary valve placement on ventricular arrhythmias. In the literature, there are few studies addressing this issue and they are all limited by small study populations (typically, less than 100 patients). An early experience reported by Therrien et al. [26] suggests that pulmonary valve replacement may reduce progression of QRS prolongation and significantly decrease the incidence of ventricular arrhythmias (from 22 to 9%) during 4.7 years of follow-up.

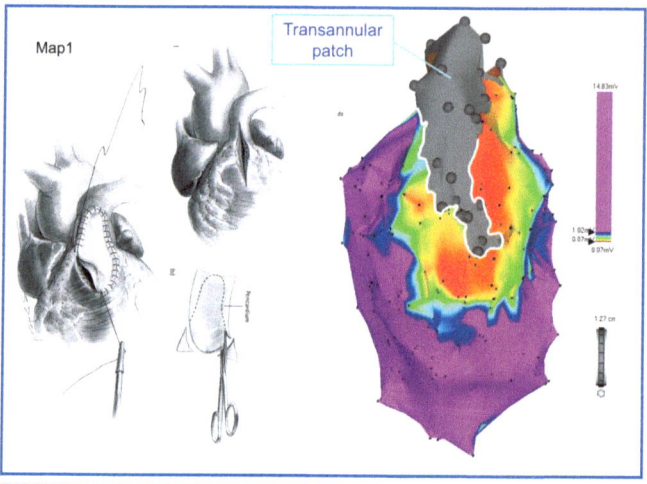

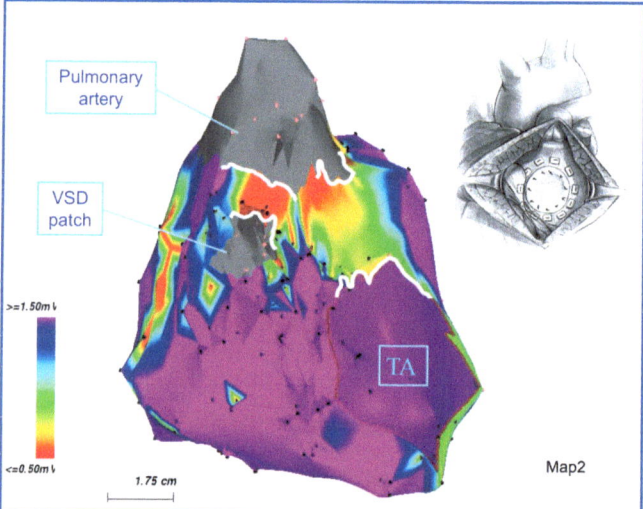

Fig. 14.5 High density contact 3D electroanatomical (EA) mapping of the RV performed during sinus rhythm identifies areas of low amplitude potentials characterized by slow conduction favouring reentrant circuit for VT. These maps were recorded in our lab, comparison with surgical anatomy is shown.

Map 1 A 3D EA map of the right ventricle obtained in a patient with severe pulmonary regurgitation and right outflow tract aneurism late after repair of TOF. The grey colour identifies the electrically silent transannular patch. Signal amplitude is shown by a colour scale; low amplitude potentials (*identified with red-yellow-green colour*) are recorded around the transannular patch and inside RVOT aneurism favouring VT reentry

Map 2 3D EA map of the RV performed during sinus rhythm in a patient who presented with VT late after repair of TOF and severe pulmonary regurgitation requiring surgery. The grey colour identifies the electrically silent VSD patch and pulmonary artery. Signal amplitude is shown by a color scale; low amplitude potentials (*identified with red-yellow-green colour*) are recorded between the pulmonary artery and the VSD patch and between the pulmonary artery and the tricuspid annulus (*TA*)

The experience published by the Boston Children's Hospital group [27] does not support a beneficial effect of pulmonary valve replacement on arrhythmia incidence. In their series, surgical treatment had no effect on VT and sudden death nor did it influence QRS duration. Noteworthy, pulmonary valve replacement in the latter study was performed when the right ventricle was severely dilated, suggesting that late correction of the hemodynamic defect cannot reverse the propensity to develop ventricular arrhythmias in these patients. In their paper, Therrien et al. [26] did not report any VT recurrence in 15 patients with ToF in whom ablation was performed at time of surgery. In the series from the Boston Children's Hospital, five of seven patients receiving cryoablation during surgery experienced VT recurrence [27].

In patient undergoing re-do surgery, the ability to reconstruct post-surgical anatomy and to identify areas of slow conduction that might sustain ventricular arrhythmias may significantly improve the efficacy of subsequent intraoperative ablation. Such a strategy, as well as the optimal timing for pulmonary valve replacement to prevent VT and sudden death, should be addressed in large multicenter studies (Fig. 14.5).

14.9   Future Perspectives

Despite considerable developments in the understanding of pathophysiology and therapeutic options, treatment and prevention of life threatening ventricular arrhythmias in adults with ToF remains an unfulfilled objective for clinicians. Close collaboration between cardiologists, surgeons and electrophysiologists is a pre-requisite for accurate identification of substrates and diagnostic paths in these patients. Multi-center collaboration on case-based therapeutic strategies will likely contribute to improve the clinical outcome of this population and significant developments are expected in the coming years.

References

1. Walsh EP, Cecchin F (2007) Arrhythmias in adult patients with congenital heart disease. Circulation 115:434-545
2. The Task Force on the Management of Grown-up Congenital Heart Disease of the European Society of Cardiology. ESC Guidelines for the management of grown-up congenital Heart Disease (new version 2010)
3. Murphy JG, Gersh BJ, Mair DD et al (1993) Long-term outcome in patients undergoing surgical repair of tetralogy of Fallot. N Engl J Med 329:593-599
4. Gatzoulis MA, Belaji S, Webber SA et al (2000) Risk factors for arrhythmia and sudden cardiac death late after repair of tetralogy of Fallot: a multicentre study. Lancet 356:875-881
5. Nollert G, Fischlein T, Bouterwek S et al (1997) Long term survival in patients with repair of tetralogy of Fallot: 36 year follow up of 490 survivors of the first year after surgical repair. J Am Coll Cardiol 30:1374-1383
6. Bouchardy J, Therrien J, Pilote L et al (2009) Atrial arrhythmias in adults with congenital heart disease. Circulation 120:1679-1686

7. Khairy P, Aboulhosn J, Gurvizet MZ et al (2010) Arrhythmia burden in adults with surgically repaired tetralogy of Fallot. A multi-institutional study. Circulation 122:868-875

8. Silka MJ, Hardy BG, Menashe VD et al (1998) A population based prospective evaluation of risk of sudden cardiac death after operation for common congenital heart defects. J Am Coll Cardiol 32:245-251

9. Friedly B, Bolens M, Taktak M et al (1988) Conduction disturbances after correction of tetralogy of Fallot: are electrophysiologic studies of prognostic value? Am Coll Cardiol 11:162-165

10. Chandar JS, Wolff GS, Garson EP (1990) Ventricular arrhythmias in post-operative tetralogy of Fallot. Am J Cardiol 65:655-661

11. Garson A, Randall DC, Gillette PC et al (1985) Prevention of sudden death after repair of tetralogy of Fallot: treatment of ventricular arrhythmias. J Am Coll Cardiol 6:221-227

12. Zahka KG, Horneffer PJ, Rowe SA et al (1988) Long-term valvular function after total repair of tetralogy of Fallot. Relation to ventricular arrhythmias. Circulation 78(Suppl 5):III14-19

13. Gatzoulis MA, Till JA, Somerville J et al (1995) Mechanoelectrical interaction in tetralogy of Fallot. Circulation 92:231-237

14. Khairy P, Landzberg MJ, Gatzoulis MA et al (2004) Value of programmed ventricular stimulation after tetralogy of Fallot repair: a multicenter study. Circulation 109:1994-2000

15. Cullen S, Celermajer DS, Franklin R et al (1994) Prognostic significance of ventricular arrhythmia after repair of tetralogy of Fallot: a 12 years prospective study. J Am Coll Cardiol 23:1151-1155

16. Hamada H, Terai M, Jibiki T et al (2002) Influence of early repair of tetralogy of Fallot without an outflow patch on late arrhythmias and sudden death: a 27 year follow-up study following a uniform surgical approach. Cardiol Young 12:345-351

17. Khairy P, Harris L, Lanzberg MJ et al (2008) Implantable cardioverter-defibrillators in tetralogy of Fallot. Circulation 117:363-370

18. Alexander ME, Walsh EP, Saul JP et al (1999) Value of programmed ventricular stimulation in patients with congenital heart disease. J Cardiovasc Electrophysiol 10:1033-1044

19. Dore A, Santagata P, Dubucet M et al (2004) Implantable cardioverter defibrillators in adults with congenital heart disease. A single center experience. PACE 27:47-51

20. Fortescue EB, Berul CI, Cecchin F et al (2004) Patient, procedural, and hardware factors associated with pacemaker lead failures in pediatrics and congenital heart disease. Heart Rhythm 1:150-159

21. Bardy GH, Smith WM, Hood MA et al (2010) An entirely subcutaneus implantable cardioverter-defibrillator. N Engl J Med 363:36-44

22. Gonska BD, Cao K, Raab J et al (1996) Radiofrequency catheter ablation of right ventricular tachycardia late after repair of congenital heart defects. Circulation 94:1902-1908

23. Furushima H, Chinushi M, Sugiura H et al (2006) Ventricular tachycardia late after repair of congenital heart disease: efficacy of combination therapy with radiofrequency catheter ablation and class III antiarrhythmic agents and long term out come. J Electrocardiol 39:219-224

24. Rostok T, Willems S, Venura R et al (2004) Radiofrequency catheter ablation of a macroreentrant ventricular tachycardia late after surgical repair of tetralogy of Fallot using the electroanatomical mapping. PACE 27:801-804

25. Zeppenfeld K, Schalji MJ, Bartelings MM et al (2007) Catheter ablation of ventricular tachycardia after repair of congenital heart disease. Electroanatomic identification of the critical right ventricular isthmus. Circulation 116:2241-2252

26. Thierrien J, Siu SC, Harris L et al (2001) Impact of pulmonary valve replacement on arrhythmia propensity late after repair of tetralogy of Fallot. Circulation 103:2489-2494

27. Harrild DM, Berul CI, Cecchi F et al (2009) Pulmonary valve replacement in tetralogy of Fallot. Impact on survival and ventricular tachycardia. Circulation 119:445-451

Perioperative Right Ventricular Management

15

Marco Ranucci

15.1 Introduction

Adults with Tetralogy of Fallot (ToF) may require surgery for a number of different reasons, the most frequent of which are (1) correction of severe pulmonary regurgitation (with or without reconstruction surgery of the dilated right ventricle (RV), (2) correction of residual defects (i.e., ventricular septal defects [VSD] or residual right ventricular outflow tract [RVOT] obstruction), and (3) complete correction of ToF in natural history or after palliation (rare in developed countries, but still common in developing countries).

Even if the physiological conditions are different in the different cases reported above, surgery of RV in the adult ToF patient is always a challenge for anesthesiologists and intensivists who take care of these complex patients. The expertise needed for correct treatment of these patients belongs to the domain of the congenital heart, and physicians used to treating pediatric congenital heart patients are probably the best choice for the perioperative treatment of these patients. However, some of the hemodynamic monitoring techniques, i.e., transesophageal echocardiography (TEE), are more commonly used in the adult cardiac surgery setting, and therefore the ideal hospital environment is that of a cardiac surgery institution treating both adult and pediatric patients.

This chapter addresses the perioperative problems in adult ToF, concentrating on the different patterns of RV perioperative pathophysiology, hemodynamic monitoring, pharmacological treatment of the failing RV, and the mechanical circulatory support of refractory RV failure.

M. Ranucci (✉)
IRCCS Policlinico San Donato, Cardio-Thoracic Anesthesia and ICU
San Donato Milanese (Mi), Italy
e-mail: cardioanestesia@virgilio.it

M. Chessa, A. Giamberti (eds.), *The Right Ventricle in Adults with Tetralogy of Fallot*,
© Springer-Verlag Italia 2012

15.2 Pathophysiological Aspects of the RV in Adult Tetralogy of Fallot

From a schematic point of view, adult ToF patients may present to the operating theater with different pathophysiologic conditions of RV function. Basically, patients scheduled for corrective surgery of a ToF in natural history have a chronic RV pressure overload that, after correction, may be converted into an acute volume overload. Conversely, patients who undergo surgery for severe pulmonary regurgitation after a previous ToF correction have a pattern of chronic volume overload. Patients requiring correction of a residual RVOT obstruction may have a mixed pattern of chronic pressure and volume overload. Finally, when the operation is required for correction of residual VSD, the hemodynamic pattern depends on the extent of the left-to-right shunt, the severity of pulmonary regurgitation, and the presence of residual RVOT obstruction.

15.2.1 Tetralogy of Fallot in Natural History or After Palliation – RV Chronic Pressure Overload

Patients who are operated in natural history or after Blalock-Taussig shunt palliation suffer from a chronic pressure overload of the RV. As a result of the RVOT obstruction, the RV is extremely hypertrophic. This pattern is always accompanied by a RV diastolic dysfunction, whereas the systolic function may be normal or decreased. Notably, it has been demonstrated that previous palliation more frequently determines an impaired systolic function of the RV. In a retrospective series of 52 adult patients who underwent total repair of ToF, Attenhofer Jost and coworkers found that patients with previous palliation had a significantly higher rate of decreased RV ejection fraction before the operation (70% vs. 4% in non-palliated patients) [1].

The diastolic dysfunction of the RV reflects the impaired relaxation of the hypertrophic myocardium, and is a right-sided equivalent of the left ventricle diastolic dysfunction observed when the left ventricular outflow tract or aortic valve are chronically obstructed.

The hemodynamic consequences of a RV diastolic dysfunction include an increased RV end diastolic pressure and increased right atrial pressure. Central venous pressure (CVP) is increased and signs of caval stasis are common, with impaired venous return mainly at the level of the inferior vena cava and visceral organs. Quantification of the RV diastolic dysfunction is based on echocardiographic measurements that are derived from those developed for the left ventricle. The transtricuspidal diastolic flow pattern may be explored using the same relative changes in E- and A-wave velocities, E/A ratios, and deceleration time as for transmitral diastolic flow in left ventricle relaxation analysis [2]. Tissue Doppler evaluation of the tricuspid valve motion may partially overcome the loading-dependent changes in transtricuspid valve diastolic flow

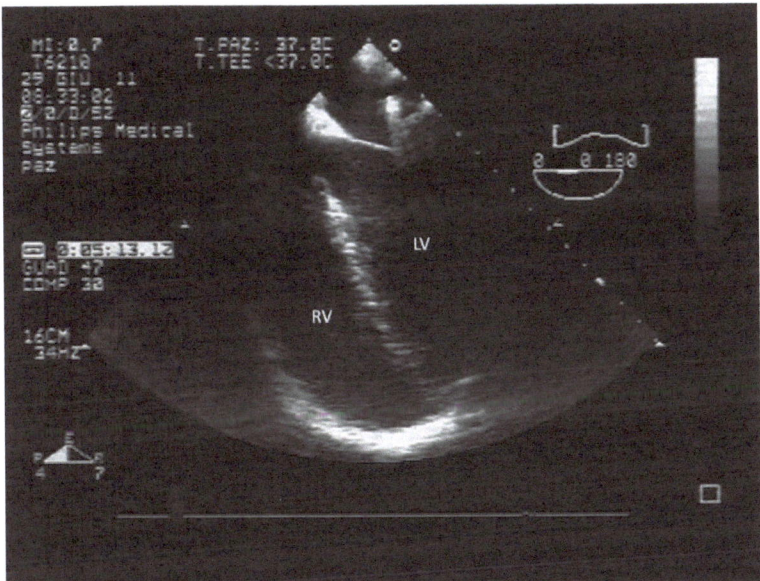

Fig. 15.1 Mid esophageal four chamber view of a dilated right ventricle (*RV*), which occupies the apex of the heart and exceeds the dimensions of the left ventricle (*LV*)

[3]. Additional information may be obtained by the analysis of the hepatic flow pattern with TEE, in analogy to the pulmonary vein flow for the left ventricle [4]. Finally, restrictive RV filling may be diagnosed in presence of a late diastolic forward flow in the pulmonary artery [5].

The hemodynamic changes after correction of ToF greatly depend on the type of correction applied to the RVOT and pulmonary valve.

Historically, different types of corrections have been applied: (1) transannular outflow patch; (2) RVOT patch with sparing of the native valve; and (3) replacement of the native pulmonary valve with or without the use of conduits.

Various series have now highlighted that adult ToF patients referred for surgical correction do not tolerate transannular patch repair well, resulting in consequent severe pulmonary regurgitation [1].

Acute and severe pulmonary regurgitation may be easily detected immediately after the repair using TEE (Figs. 15.1, 15.2) color-flow Doppler and continuous wave (CW) Doppler. The presence of an acute pulmonary regurgitation causes a further deterioration of diastolic RV function. Diastolic filling of the RV is already impaired by the hypertrophic myocardial conditions, and the retrograde diastolic filling of the RV due to the pulmonary regurgitation further impairs the ability of the RV to recruit volume through the pulmonary circulation into the systemic circulation.

Patients with this pattern often experience a postoperative low cardiac output syndrome (LCOS) and are more prone to subsequent operations (pulmonary valve replacement) [1, 6, 7].

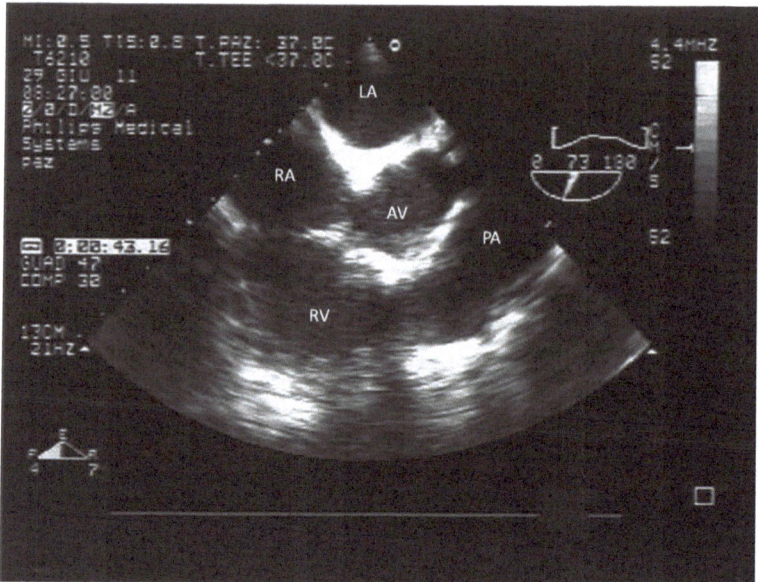

Fig. 15.2 Inflow-outflow view of the right ventricle (*RV*) with the aortic valve (*AV*), the right atrium (*RA*), the left atrium (*LA*), and the pulmonary artery (*PA*)

15.2.2 Reoperation of Adult Tetralogy of Fallot Patients with Severe Pulmonary Regurgitation – the Chronic Volume Overload

The history of ToF repair with transannular patch in the pediatric age is burdened by the problem of pulmonary valve regurgitation, RV dilation and dysfunction, and aneurysm of the RVOT patch [8–15].

The progressive volume overload determines a deterioration of the systolic function of the RV. At the transthoracic echo (TTE) examination or transesophageal echocardiogram (TEE) the systolic function of the RV can be addressed with techniques that differ from the assessment of left ventricular function. Due to its elliptical shape that cannot be easily translated into a solid geometrical volume, the RV ejection fraction is rarely used. Tricuspid annular plane systolic excursion (TAPSE) quantifies the movement of the lateral tricuspid valve annulus towards the RV apex during systole. This measurement overcomes the problems related to the difficult geometry of the RV, and correlates well with the angiographically determined RV ejection fraction [16]. Normal values of TAPSE are around 25 mm, and severe RV systolic function may be diagnosed when TAPSE is less than 12–14 mm.

Since the RV contractility greatly depends on the free wall movement, a M-Mode study of the free wall excursion may be done with either TTE or TEE (in the inflow-outflow view). Other more complex assessments of the systolic

RV function include the total ejection isovolume (TEI) index and tissue velocity, strain, and strain rate with tissue Doppler.

Patients previously operated on for ToF may demonstrate a systolic dysfunction of the left ventricle [17], which appears not to be related to the severity of pulmonary regurgitation. Conversely, systolic RV dysfunction appears significantly associated with systolic left ventricular dysfunction [18]. Both pressure and volume overload of the RV ventricle have deleterious reflections on left ventricular systolic function: the mechanical interaction of the two ventricles is even enhanced by the presence of septal defect patch. Other mechanisms that link the RV and left ventricular function are electrical dyssynchrony and neurohormonal coupling.

15.3   Perioperative Monitoring of RV Function

Monitoring of the adult ToF patient who requires a cardiac operation includes many of the available tools routinely used in cardiac operations, plus additional techniques of specific interest for the RV function assessment.

A central venous catheter is mandatory for the continuous measurement of the CVP. Both systolic and diastolic dysfunction of the RV are accompanied by elevated values of CVP, and the morphology of the CVP signal may allow detection of the existence and severity of tricuspid regurgitation. Tricuspid regurgitation is common in adult patients with repaired ToF, due to the already mentioned progressive and chronic volume overload and RV dilatation. CVP measurement may guide fluid administration and allows assessment of the efficacy of vasoactive drugs used to sustain the contractility of the failing RV.

Pulmonary artery catheters (PAC) could theoretically offer valuable hemodynamic information in patients with a RV dysfunction or failure. Apart from the measurement of cardiac output, they provide a direct assessment of the right-sided heart pressures (CVP and pulmonary artery pressure). Moreover, specific PACs are now available, equipped with an algorithm for the determination of the RV end-diastolic volume and ejection fraction [19].

However, in the specific setting of the adult patient who requires an operation on the RV and/or pulmonary valve, the role of PACs appears very limited. The presence of a usually at least moderate tricuspid regurgitation and pulmonary regurgitation makes the RV end diastolic volume and ejection fraction calculations unreliable [20]. The need to operate on the right heart chambers makes the positioning of the PAC an obstacle for the surgeon's maneuvers. Finally, the use of patches, conduits, and prosthetic valves on right heart chambers makes a long-permanence PAC a threat for infections.

As an adjunct to the standard CVC, it is reasonable to use oxymetric catheters which can provide a continuous measurement of the central venous oxygen saturation (SvO_2). SvO_2 provides reliable information about the adequacy of the cardiac output with respect to the metabolic needs, and may guide diagnosis and treatment in case of perioperative RV failure.

A central role in the hemodynamic monitoring of the adult ToF patient is played by the TEE. The RV and its hemodynamic measurements may be studied using four standard TEE views. The mid-esophageal, four chamber view allows detection of the border of the RV, and its relationship with the left ventricle (Fig. 15.1). The hypertrophic RV appears as a structure with a greatly enhanced myocardial wall, whereas the dilated RV loses its natural elliptic shape and occupies the apex of the heart. The subaortic ventricular septal defect or the defect patch may be appreciated in this view. From this position, by simply shifting to a 45°C view, the RV inflow-outflow view is obtained. This image (Fig. 15.2) is of paramount importance, because it includes many of the typical findings of ToF. The RV is visible as a structure that embraces the aortic valve (in short axis in the middle of the screen), with the tricuspid valve on the left side (inflow) and the pulmonary valve and artery on the right side (outflow) of the screen. The RV free wall (at the bottom of the screen) may be appreciated for its movement and excursion using an M-Mode analysis.

The tricuspid valve can be explored for TAPSE in this view, and in presence of tricuspid valve regurgitation. This is one of the best views for obtaining a parallelism with the regurgitant flow and therefore measuring the systolic pulmonary pressure with a CW Doppler. Finally, this is the best views for appreciating the extent and position of the RVOT obstruction (Fig. 15.2).

The anatomy of the pulmonary valve and artery may be appreciated using an upper esophageal aortic arch short axis view. In this image (Fig. 15.3) the final part of the aortic arch is located at the top of the screen, with the left subclavian artery visible, and on the left side of the screen there is the long axis view of the pulmonary artery and valve. In this position, it is very easy to obtain a perfect parallelism and to assess the degree of the transpulmonary gradient and pulmonary regurgitation using a color Doppler and a CW Doppler study.

Finally, inserting the probe into the stomach, the transgastric view is obtained. In this position the left ventricle is on the right side of the screen, and the right ventricle on the left. The ratio between the two ventricles' volume may be assessed, and it is possible to obtain again a good parallel with the transpulmonary flow, measuring the systolic gradient and the diastolic regurgitant flow (Fig. 15.4).

Other hemodynamic monitoring tools may be useful in case of perioperative RV failure. Arterial waveform pulse contour analysis systems may be used for obtaining an estimate of the cardiac output and of the left ventricular filling status (derived from the systolic pressure variation). Near infrared spectroscopy can provide a continuous indirect estimate of the cerebral SvO_2 and serial blood lactate determination may provide information related to the adequacy of the cardiac output with respect to the metabolic needs.

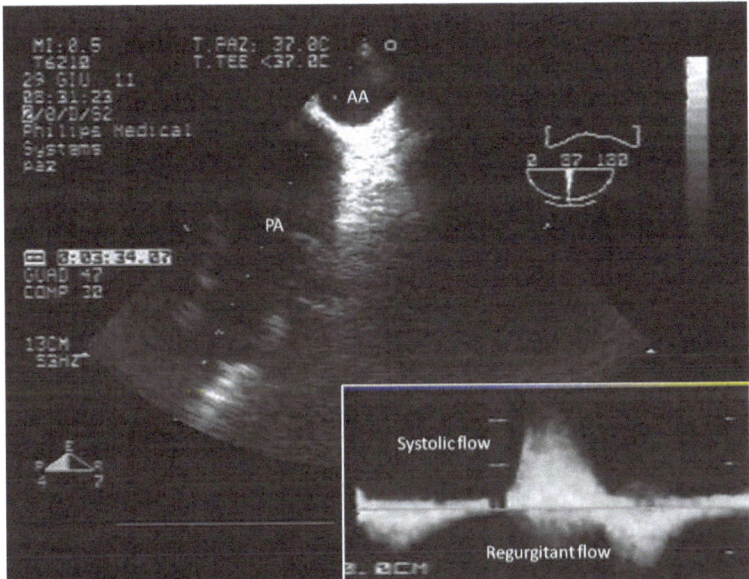

Fig. 15.3 Upper esophageal aortic arch (*AA*) short axis view for the Doppler study of the pulmonary artery (*PA*) flow

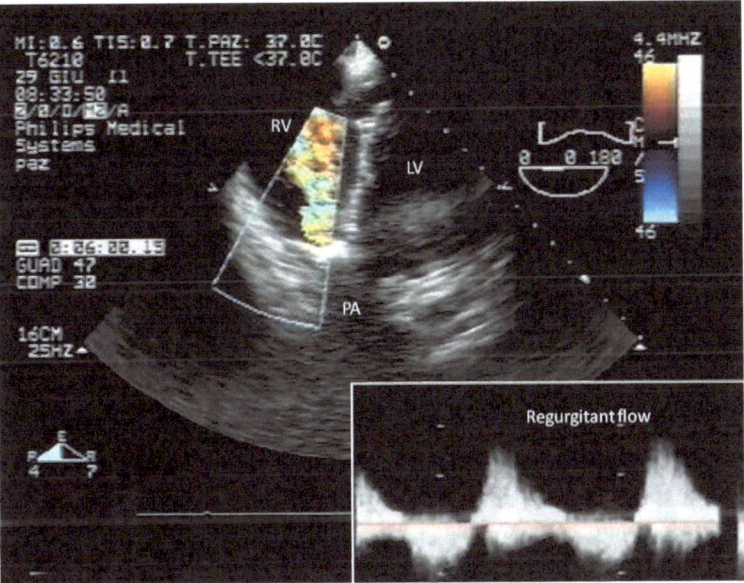

Fig. 15.4 Transgastric view of the right ventricle (*RV*), pulmonary artery (*PA*), regurgitant pulmonary valve and left ventricle (*LV*), with the Doppler study of the transpulmonary flow

15.4 The Failing Right Ventricle

Adult patients receiving complete Fallot correction or additional procedures after a previous complete correction may experience acute right ventricular failure after the operation. This pattern may appear immediately after completion of the operation in the theatre, or in the first postoperative hours in the intensive care unit. The basic pathophysiological mechanisms recognize the preoperative diastolic and/or systolic dysfunction, which may deteriorate due to the ischemia-reperfusion insult during the operation. The hypertrophic right ventricle may be difficult to protect during the ischemic time of the aortic cross-clamping, despite the use of adequate cardioplegic solutions. The hemodynamic marker of the RV failure is the inability of the RV to recruit volume into the systemic circulation. Under these conditions, the clinical pattern is quite specific: the left ventricle appears unloaded, with all the dynamic fluid responsiveness indicators (pulse pressure variation, systolic pressure variation) suggestive of a hypovolemic condition. Actually, rather than being an absolute hypovolemia, this condition is a relative hypovolemia of the systemic circulation, with a large amount of unrecruitable fluids placed in the venous bed.

As a result, the CVP is high (> 15 mmHg) and the inferior vena cava and hepatic veins are overloaded. The right ventricle may appear dilated in case of systolic dysfunction with pulmonary regurgitation, or hypertrophic with a reduced end diastolic volume in the restrictive diastolic pattern.

The global cardiac output is inadequate, with reduced systemic arterial pressure, urine output, SvO_2 (< 68%), and increased arterial serum lactates (> 3 mMol/L). The end-tidal CO_2 is typically reduced, as an expression of a reduced pulmonary blood flow, and a large venous-arterial CO_2 gradient may appear.

15.4.1 Pharmacological Strategies for the Treatment of Acute RV Failure

Different drugs may be used for the treatment of the failing RV, and many therapeutic algorithms greatly depend on the physician's preference. However, there is a general agreement on the use of the phopshodiesterase inhibitor milrinone (dose 0.375–0.75 µg/kg/min). This drug may be particularly useful for the treatment of systolic dysfunction, without deteriorating the diastolic function due to its action which is independent on adrenoreceptor activity. Milrinone seems to improve myocardial relaxation and induces a limited increase in myocardial oxygen demands. Its role in the treatment of acute heart failure following pediatric cardiac surgery is well established [21, 22]. However, it must be considered that milrinone induces a considerable systemic vasodilation, and its effects should be considered within a comprehensive strategy of RV preload preservation. In this respect, the patients with RV diastolic dysfunction and no left ventricular dysfunction may benefit from a moderate systemic vasoconstriction (norepinephrine, 0.05–0.2 µg/kg/min).

When milrinone alone is insufficient, direct adrenoreceptor agents may be added, like dopamine (3–8 mcg/kg/min) or epinephrine (0.02–0.2 mcg/kg/min). Both these agents increase the heart rate and may be responsible for arrhythmias. Information of the efficacy of new generation inotropic agents (levosimendan) is anecdotal and not supported, at present, by the existing literature.

15.4.2 Non-pharmacological Strategies for the Treatment of Acute RV Failure

The failing RV needs an appropriate preload to recruit blood from the venous system towards the systemic circulation. Therefore, CVP values in the range of 12–15 mmHg are not unusual and may be required.

Diastolic filling should be facilitated by guaranteeing correct atrio-ventricular conduction and a normal heart rate. Tachycardia decreases the diastolic filling time, and junctional rhythm or any pattern of atrio-ventricular block exclude the atrial contribution to the diastolic filling. Therefore, the use of atrio-ventricular pacing is mandatory in the absence of a spontaneous normal conduction and heart rate.

The heart-lung interaction under mechanical ventilation is of particular importance in the setting of an impaired blood transit through the pulmonary vessels. Positive pressure ventilation decreases venous return, RV preload and cardiac output, especially when a positive end-respiratory pressure is applied. At the same time, pulmonary vessel compression during positive pressure ventilation increases the RV afterload. Mechanical ventilation should therefore be settled at the lowest possible positive pressure regimen, however avoiding the occurrence of hypoxia and/or hypercapnia, which determine pulmonary vasoconstriction.

Inhaled nitric oxide (iNO) is a powerful pulmonary arterial vasodilator. Its role in congenital heart surgery is limited to the treatment of pulmonary hypertension and is of course absent in the treatment of the ToF. However, some patients who received a Blalock-Taussig palliation may have areas of inhomogeneous pulmonary blood flow after correction, and anecdotal reports of the use of iNO in the treatment of RV failure exist [23].

RV failure refractory to pharmacological treatment may require additional measures, ranging from the need for leaving an open sternum, to mechanical circulatory support. Even if the primary culprit for the low cardiac output state is RV failure, isolated RV assistance is difficult to perform, due to the need for pulmonary artery cannulation and the presence of different degrees of residual pulmonary regurgitation. Therefore, mechanical assistance of the failing RV in the adult ToF is based on the placement of an extracorporeal membrane oxygenation (ECMO) system. This includes a venous and arterial cannulation, a centrifugal pump, an oxygenator and a heat-exchanger. Depending on the situation, the cannulas can be directly inserted into the right atrium and the ascending aorta when the chest is open, or through the groin (femoral vein and artery) once it is closed. ECMO in refractory RV failure after cardiac operations in adult ToF patients should be considered a bridge-to-recovery or a bridge-to-transplant, depending on the clinical characteristics of the patient.

References

1. Attenhofer Jost CH, Connolly HM, Burkhart HM et al (2010) Tetralogy of Fallot repair in patients 40 years or older. Mayo Clin Proc 85:1090-1094
2. Spencer KT, Weinert L, Lang RM (1999) Effect of age, heart rate and tricuspid regurgitation on the Doppler echocardiographic evaluation of right ventricular diastolic function. Cardiology 92:59-64
3. Cicala S, Galderisi M, Caso P et al (2002) Right ventricular diastolic dysfunction in arterial systemic hypertension: analysis by pulsed tissue Doppler. Eur J Echocardiogr 3:135-142
4. Nomura T, Lebowitz L, Koide Y et al (1995) Evaluation of hepatic venous flow using transesophageal echocardiography in coronary artery bypass surgery: an index of right ventricular function. J Cardiothorac Vasc Anesth 9:9-17
5. Gatzoulis MA, Clark AL, Cullen S et al (1995) Right ventricular diastolic function 15 to 35 years after repair of tetralogy of Fallot: restrictive physiology predicts superior exercise performance. Circulation 91:1775-1781
6. Bacha EA, Scheule AM, Zurakowski D et al (2001) Long-term results after early primary repair of tetralogy of Fallot. J Thorac Cardiovasc Surg 122:154-161
7. Erdogan HB, Bozbuga N, Kayalar N et al (2005) Long-term outcome after total correction of tetralogy of Fallot in adolescent and adult age. J Card Surg 20:119-123
8. Waien SA, Liu PP, Ross BL et al (1992) Serial follow-up of adults with repaired tetralogy of Fallot. J Am Coll Cardiol 20:295-300
9. Oechslin EN, Harrison DA, Harris L et al (1999) Reoperation in adults with repair of tetralogy of Fallot: indications and outcomes. J Thorac Cardiovasc Surg 118:245-251
10. Discigil B, Dearani JA, Puga FJ et al (2001) Late pulmonary valve replacement after repair of tetralogy of Fallot. J Thorac Cardiovasc Surg 121:344-351
11. de Ruijter FT, Weenink I, Hitchcock FJ et al (2002) Right ventricular dysfunction and pulmonary valve replacement after correction of tetralogy of Fallot. Ann Thorac Surg 73:1794-1800
12. Therrien J, Siu SC, McLaughlin PR et al (2000) Pulmonary valve replacement in adults late after repair of tetralogy of Fallot: are we operating too late? J Am Coll Cardiol 36:1670-1675
13. Davlouros PA, Karatza AA, Gatzoulis MA, Shore DF (2004) Timing and type of surgery for severe pulmonary regurgitation after repair of tetralogy of Fallot. Int J Cardiol 97(Suppl. 1):91-101
14. D'Udekem Y, Pasquet A, Van Caenegem O et al (2004) Reoperation for severe right ventricular dilatation after tetralogy of Fallot repair: pulmonary infundibuloplasty should be added to homograft implantation. J Heart Valve Dis 13:307-312
15. D'Udekem Y, Rubay J, Ovaert C (2001) Failure of right ventricular recovery of Fallot patients after pulmonary valve replacement: delay of reoperation or surgical technique? J Am Coll Cardiol 37:2008-2009
16. Kaul S, Tei C, Hopkins JM, Shah PM (1984) Assessment of right ventricular function using two-dimensional echocardiography. Am Heart J 107:526-531
17. Broberg CS, Aboulhosn J, Mongeon F-P et al (2011) Prevalence of left ventricular systolic dysfunction in adults with repaired Tetralogy of Fallot. Am J Cardiol 107: 1215-1220
18. Davlouros PA, Kilner PJ, Hornung TS et al (2001) Right ventricular function in adults with repaired tetralogy of Fallot assessed with cardiovascular magnetic resonance imaging: detrimental role of right ventricular outflow aneurysms or akinesia and adverse right-to-left ventricular interaction. J Am Coll Cardiol 40:2044-2052

19. Ranucci M (2006) Which cardiac surgical patients can benefit from placement of a pulmonary artery catheter? Crit Care 10 (suppl 3):S6
20. Spinale FG, Mukherjee R, Tanaka R, Zile MR (1992) The effects of valvular regurgitation on thermodilution ejection fraction measurements. Chest 101:723-731
21. Hoffman TM, Wernovsky G, Atz AM et al (2003) Efficacy and safety of milrinone in preventing low cardiac output syndrome in infants and children after corrective surgery for congenital heart disease. Circulation 107:996-1002
22. Chang AC, Atz AM, Wernovsky G et al (1995) Milrinone: systemic and pulmonary hemodynamic effects in neonates after cardiac surgery. Crit Care Med 23:1907-1914
23. Booker BD, Prosser DP, Franks R et al (1996) Nitric oxide in the treatment of acute right ventricular failure after surgical correction of tetralogy of Fallot. J Cardiothorac Vasc Anesth 10:973-974

Subject Index

22q11.2 deletion syndrome 31
8p23 deletion 29, 31

A
Abnormal morphology of the septo-parietal
   bands 6
Absence of the pulmonary valve cusps 20
Accessory atrioventricular tissue 11
Acute right ventricular failure 186
Acute volume overload 180
Additional muscular 11-12
Adult congenital heart disease (ACHD) 1, 57,
   145, 155-156, 159, 167, 173
Alagille syndrome 30, 32-34
Anomalies of the mitral valve 11
Anti-arrhythmic drug therapy 173, 175
Aortic overriding 4, 9-10
Arterial duct 13
Atrial septal defect (ASD) 28, 107, 133, 149,
   156, 162

B
Bone marrow cell 42

C
c-kit 41-42
Cardiac catheterization 92, 96, 117, 138, 157
Cardiac Magnetic Resonance (CMR) 79-85,
   116-117
Cardiac regeneration 41, 43
Cardiac stem cells (CSCs) 39, 41-44
Cardio pulmonary exercise test (CPET) 109
Central venous catheter 183
CHARGE syndrome 30, 32
Chest x-ray 81, 115
Chromosome 16, 31
Chronic pressure overload 53, 180
Chronic volume overload 52, 77, 96, 159,

   180, 182-183
Collateral systemic-to-pulmonary arteries 10-
   11, 16
Color Flow Doppler 181,
Computerized tomography (CT) 117
Congenital heart disease (ACHD) 1, 20, 43,
   47, 53, 56-57, 61, 78, 82, 133, 137, 155,
   163, 167
Coronary arteries 16, 21, 72, 75
Crista supraventricularis 4-5

D
Diagnosis 2, 35, 130, 183
Diastolic dysfunction 78, 94-95, 109, 116,
   172, 180, 183, 186
Differentiation 28, 41-44, 48
Dilatation of the aortic root 13
Dopamine 187
Double aortic arch 13, 15, 20-21

E
ECG-recording 92
Echocardiography 56, 68, 70, 80, 82, 85, 92,
   96, 101-102, 115, 130, 138, 145, 149, 179
Electrophysiological study 145, 169
Embryonic stem cells 40
Epinephrine 187
Exercise studies 116
Extra cardiac anomalies 16, 22
Extracorporeal membrane oxygenation
   (ECMO) 187-188

F
Fractional Area Change (FAC) 101-102

G
Gene
   FOG2 gene 33

JAG1 gene 30, 32-33, 35
NKX2.5 gene 28, 32-33, 41-42
TBX1 gene 31, 33, 48

H
Heart
    failure 39-40, 42-43, 53-54, 56-57, 64, 66,
    78, 81, 114, 131, 156, 186
    surgery 64, 187

I
Index of Myocardial Performance (IMP) 103
Induced Pluripotent Stem Cells (iPSCs) 40
Inflow 4, 50, 82, 91, 101, 182, 184
Implantable cardioverter defibrillator 71
Intensive care unit 138, 186
Isovolumic acceleration time 104-105

L
Landmark 5-6, 13
Levosimendan 187
Longitudinal and radial strain and SR 105

M
Mid-esophageal, four chamber view 184
Milrinone 186-187
Moderator band 4-5, 16, 50-51
MRI volumes measurement 92, 94, 100, 103,
    117, 119, 121, 145
Muscular infundibular ventricular defect 9

N
Nitric oxide 187
Nuclear cardiology studies 117

O
Oculo-Auriculo-Vertebral Spectrum
    (Goldenhar syndrome) 30, 32
Origin of the left subclavian 13
Outflow 19, 27-28, 48,66, 78, 91, 115, 121,
    131, 139,148, 169-170, 174, 176, 182,
    184
    right ventricular outflow 4-5, 7, 9, 11, 13,
    16-17, 50-52, 54, 56-57, 61, 75, 101, 114,
    118, 119, 127, 129, 138, 145, 157, 179
    left ventricular outflow 5, 11, 12, 51, 139,
    148, 180
    pulmonary outflow 19, 50, 66

P
Perimembranous ventricular septal defect 9-
    11, 18-19
Pressure Half Time 93, 116

Pressure overload 52-53, 55, 75-76, 100, 168,
    180
Pulmonary
    atresia (PA) 4, 7, 10-11, 16, 19-20, 28-29,
    31, 34, 62, 128, 130
    regurgitation 13, 17, 52, 54-56, 69-70, 76-
    78, 81-82, 91-96, 104, 113, 116, 119-121,
    131, 149, 157, 176, 179-184, 186-187
    stenosis 3-4, 6-7, 13, 16-17, 19, 28, 32, 50,
    62, 91, 96, 120, 134, 145, 147-148
Pulmonary valve
    dysfunction 131, 148
    implantation 2, 120, 145-146, 150-151, 160
    replacement (PVR) 1, 56, 63, 69, 78, 92, 113,
    117, 119-121, 145, 148, 155, 175, 177, 181

Q
Quantification of pulmonary regurgitation 93,
    113

R
Re-intervention 68, 91, 175
Recombinant 8 syndrome 31
Recurrence risk 34
Recruit 181, 186-187
Regenerating 39
Reprogramming 40-41, 53
Restrictive right ventricle 94-95
Retro esophageal course of the right subcla-
    vian artery 13
Reversine 40-41
Right aortic arch 13-14, 16, 20-21, 49, 163
Right ventricle 3-4, 6, 9-10, 12, 16, 19, 28-29,
    39, 43-44, 47-57, 70, 75, 78-79, 84-85, 91,
    94-95, 100-102, 104, 107, 109, 114, 119,
    121, 125, 128-131, 138-141, 146, 150, 170,
    172, 176-177, 179, 181-182, 184-186
Right ventricular (RV)
    function 53, 55-56, 71, 85, 91-92, 100, 105,
    109, 129, 131, 159
    volumes 92, 115, 117, 120, 131
Risk stratification 169, 171-172
RV inflow-outflow view 184
RVOT Morphology 95, 145-146, 149

S
Secondary heart field 27-28, 34, 48-49
Septo-parietal bands 5-7, 17
Stem cell
    bone marrow stem cells 42
    cardiac stem cells (CSCs) 39, 41, 43-44
    induced pluripotent stem cells (iPSCs) 40
    mesenchymal stem cells (MSCs) 42
    stem cell niches 39

Stenosis of the pulmonary arteries 14
Strain rate (SR) 82, 85, 105, 183
Straddling or overriding tricuspid valve 9, 11
Sudden death 16, 19, 44, 54, 57, 63, 69, 81, 92, 115-117, 131, 134, 160, 169, 171-172, 174-175, 177
Subarterial 3, 8-9, 16
Surgical anatomy 168, 174, 176-177
Syndrome
    Down syndrome 11, 28-29, 34
    Low cardiac output syndrome (LCOS) 181
Systolic function

T
Three dimensional echocardiography
Timing for reintervention
ToF surgical correction
Trabecula septomarginalis
Transcatheter ablation
Transesophageal Echocardiography (TEE) 138, 141, 179, 181-182, 184
Transgastric view 184-185
Transthoracic echocardiographic (TTE) and Doppler assessment 115
Treatment 2, 35, 40-42, 44, 61, 65, 69, 91, 117, 119, 125-126, 128, 131, 133, 135, 146,

158-162, 169, 175, 177, 179, 183, 186-187
Trisomy 13 21-22, 28-29
Trisomy 18 21-22, 28-29
Trisomy 21 (Down syndrome) 20-22, 28-29, 34, 43
Two chambered right ventricle 16

U
Umbilical cord blood mononuclear cell (UCMNC) 44
Unrecruitable 186
Upper esophageal aortic arch short axis view 184

V
VACTERL Association 30, 32, 34
Ventricular
    arrhythmias 1, 81, 114-115, 117, 120-121, 134, 145-146, 155, 160-161, 167-170, 172, 174-175, 177
    remodeling 47, 52-53, 55-56
    septal defect (VSD) 3-4, 6, 8-12, 18-19, 21, 28, 30-31, 50-52, 54, 66, 75, 133, 138, 141, 149, 156, 169, 179, 184
    tachycardia (VT) 54, 57, 84, 160-162, 167, 174